"I've a better idea. How about we go for a meal later on?"

It was a lovely thought, even though it meant something more personal than walking in the hills. Or did it? Was she overreacting to a simple invitation to have dinner together? Probably, but then that's what she did. "I'd like that. A lot," she added without thought, and didn't regret it for a moment. It would be fun to go out with a man who had her heating up one moment, then cooling off the next as reality set in. Shaun was opening her eyes to a new world, and whatever the outcome, she was going to grab the moments they had together and make the most of whatever was on offer. Dinner was dinner, no more, no less. It could be a lot more. *Stop it. You've said yes, so make the most of it and see where this new friendship goes from here.*

Dear Reader,

When a bus runs into people, chaos ensues in the Emergency department where Nikki and Shaun are on duty. It is Shaun's first week working there and Nikki knows he's very good at his job.

But it's when he stands by her when the reporters start asking about their patients that she begins to see him in a different light. She's known for her bravery by jumping in front of a racing car to grab and save a wee boy who'd run away from his mother, and the reporters expect her to talk about the people injured by the bus.

Shaun isn't recognized from when he brought a plane down after the pilot, his best friend, died midair.

Since Nikki's husband left her at a vulnerable time, she's not ready to trust her heart again. Neither is Shaun after the ramifications of losing his mate, then his wife.

Can these two work through the barriers they've erected around themselves and find true love?

I hope you enjoy reading their story and seeing how Nikki and Shaun move on with their lives.

All the best,

Sue MacKay

A FLING WITH THE ER DOC

SUE MacKAY

Harlequin

MEDICAL ROMANCE

![H] Harlequin®
MEDICAL
ROMANCE

ISBN-13: 978-1-335-99346-5

A Fling with the ER Doc

Harlequin Enterprises ULC
22 Adelaide St. West, 41st Floor
Toronto, Ontario M5H 4E3, Canada
www.Harlequin.com

HarperCollins Publishers
Macken House, 39/40 Mayor Street Upper,
Dublin 1, D01 C9W8, Ireland
www.HarperCollins.com

Printed in U.S.A.

Sue MacKay lives with her husband in New Zealand's beautiful Marlborough Sounds, with the water on her doorstep and the birds and the trees at her back door. It is the perfect setting to indulge her passions of entertaining friends by cooking them sumptuous meals, drinking fabulous wine, going for hill walks or kayaking around the bay—and, of course, writing stories.

Books by Sue MacKay

Harlequin Medical Romance

Stranded with the Paramedic
Single Mom's New Year Wish
Brought Together by a Pup
Fake Fiancée to Forever?
Resisting the Pregnant Pediatrician
Marriage Reunion with the Island Doc
Paramedic's Fling to Forever
Healing the Single Dad Surgeon
Brooding Vet for the Wallflower
Wedding Date with the ER Doctor
Parisian Surgeon's Secret Child

Visit the Author Profile page
at Harlequin.com for more titles.

CHAPTER ONE

'SHAUN, I NEED you here. Now.' Emergency doctor Nikki Marlow didn't wait for a reply, if there was one coming. Instead, she got on with making an incision to insert a tube into the chest of the woman writhing in agony on the board in front her. 'Pneumothorax. I concur with the paramedic's diagnosis of fractured ribs being the cause.'

'Tell me when you're ready and I'll insert the tube,' Dr Shaun Elliott said as he joined Nikki. Running a hand down the woman's right side to her pelvis and lower to her hips, he reported back. 'More injuries here.'

'I'm making the incision between the third and fourth ribs.' As she cut in, a nurse swabbed the site. Then it was done, and she held the incision open and nodded at Shaun.

'Here we go.' His fingers firmly pushed the tube through the incision, then stopped. He turned the tube further to the right, pressed again, and it went into place. 'I'll hold it while you stitch it.'

Nikki took a threaded needle from the nurse

CHAPTER ONE

'SHAUN, I NEED you here. Now.' Emergency doctor Nikki Marlow didn't wait for a reply, if there was one coming. Instead, she got on with making an incision to insert a tube into the chest of the woman writhing in agony on the board in front her. 'Pneumothorax. I concur with the paramedic's diagnosis of fractured ribs being the cause.'

'Tell me when you're ready and I'll insert the tube,' Dr Shaun Elliott said as he joined Nikki. Running a hand down the woman's right side to her pelvis and lower to her hips, he reported back. 'More injuries here.'

'I'm making the incision between the third and fourth ribs.' As she cut in, a nurse swabbed the site. Then it was done, and she held the incision open and nodded at Shaun.

'Here we go.' His fingers firmly pushed the tube through the incision, then stopped. He turned the tube further to the right, pressed again, and it went into place. 'I'll hold it while you stitch it.'

Nikki took a threaded needle from the nurse

standing opposite her. 'Thanks, Georgie.' As she worked, she asked Shaun, 'Do you think there're more fractures elsewhere?'

'Her pelvis feels soft, as if it's been shattered, plus I'm not sure her hip's in much better shape.'

'I'll call radiology as soon as I'm done here, and also let the surgical unit know the first patient's ready and needs to be taken to Theatre to deal with the pneumothorax before anything else.'

'Want me here, or should I attend the patient who's being placed on the next bed? He's got fractured femurs and abdominal injuries.'

The second victim had arrived. Two down, five to come, and those were only the seriously injured. Nikki shuddered at the thought of a bus careering into pedestrians on a crossing. An image that kept her awake many nights flicked across her mind. A small boy running away from his mum onto a busy city road right in front of a speeding car. Hideous. Terrifying. 'Yes, Shaun, you go to him. Take Sarah with you.' The junior doctor looked pale but determined to deal with whatever was required in the coming hours. 'Sarah, do as Shaun says and you'll be fine.'

Sarah flicked her a tight look. 'Of course.'

Shaun gave them both a smile. 'We've got this.'

'I know we have.' Nikki ignored the stunning smile that the new doctor turned on easily and focused on her patient, leaving the other two to get on with theirs. The woman's abdomen was

swollen, probably from an internal haemorrhage.
'I need a phone—'

'I'm here.' A surgeon spoke from right behind
her. 'Pneumothorax, I heard. Fill me in on everything.'

Nikki gave him a relieved smile. 'Unconfirmed
fractured ribs, punctured lungs. Haven't had time
to arrange radiology. The pelvis appears badly
fractured, as does her hip. Her abdomen's swollen.'

The surgeon was checking the monitor, assessing the low oxygen levels and increased heart
rate. 'Leave her with me. I'll get her into Theatre
and arrange radiology. You've got plenty going
on without this one.'

They sure did. 'Thanks, Jack.' Nikki looked
around and saw paramedics wheeling in another
patient with an ED doctor on hand. The department was filling up fast. It seemed only minutes
ago she'd informed the staff about what was coming, and everyone had been quick to prepare. Radiology and Theatre had also been warned. The
unfortunate patients who'd come to the emergency department prior to the call saying to expect numerous code-five patients could be sitting
in the waiting room for hours to come. They
might be ill, but serious impact injuries came
before most other cases. As far as she knew, no
one out there was a code five. The triage nurse
would've told her.

Leaving Jack with the woman, Nikki crossed over to Shaun and his patient. 'Fill me in.'

'Not good.' Shaun glanced up at her, anguish filling his eyes, before turning back to the heart monitor.

Dark blue eyes, Nikki suddenly noted. She shook her head. Out of order. She was in the middle of an emergency. What did it matter what colour his eyes were? 'Tell me more.'

'He arrested on the way in. The paramedics revived him. Then he had a second event here as he was being rolled out of the ambulance. His heart rate's so low, I'm surprised it's beating at all.'

'Serious head injury.' She carefully touched the man's scalp. 'Blunt force trauma.' She shook her head. This was awful. What had the bus driver been doing to not stop for people on a controlled crossing?

'Here we go again,' Shaun said as the heart monitor flatlined. 'Stand back.' After quickly checking everyone had moved out of touch of the bed and patient, he gave the man an electric shock.

Nikki held her breath, her eyes fixed on the monitor. The line wobbled, returned to flat.

'Again.' Shaun looked determined this man was going to make it no matter what, like he was going to personally ensure the man's heart restarted and stayed beating.

Something she understood too well. After saving that little boy, Jordie, who tore out onto the road, she knew too well how fragile life could be. 'Go, Shaun,' she muttered under her breath.

'Doing all I can.'

So much for thinking she'd spoken to herself. Sometimes in this job it didn't hurt to let people know how you felt about their work though. Everyone would be pulling out all stops to get the best results for the people being brought in from the accident, but she'd never seen someone quite so determined as Shaun to get a stopped heart beating. A bad experience in his past? Staring at the screen, she saw when the next shock slammed into the man's body. Saw the green line move in the right directions—up, then down. Up, then down. 'Phew.' As she glanced around the department, her relief disappeared. More ambulance gurneys were being pushed into the room. Numerous paramedics were talking to other doctors and nurses about their patients. 'Kennedy,' she called to one of the doctors. 'Can you prioritise? Shaun needs another pair of hands here.' Prioritising was her role, but Kennedy wasn't new to it.

'No problem.'

Shaun said, 'Nikki, can you deal with the head injury while I look after the heart problem and check out the cause of massive bruising in his groin?' He didn't wait for an answer. 'Sarah, the left knee appears dislocated.'

The list of injuries seemed endless. Nikki

in here by ambulance.' She glanced at the paramedic, one eyebrow raised.

'A policewoman's bringing Sammy in. He's got lots of bruising to his arms and legs but otherwise appears to have escaped any serious injuries. Of course an X-ray will confirm that.'

'I don't care,' Carol cried. 'I want him checked out by a doctor.'

Ouch. Paramedics were very good at their jobs. They faced trauma most days. 'Carol, take a deep breath.' The woman was in shock, and the fact her son had been hurt even mildly would add to the stress going on in her head. 'The paramedics know what they're doing just as well as the doctors in here. If this man says your lad has dodged serious injuries, then you can believe him.'

Carol stared at her with wide eyes. 'I'm so worried,' she said more quietly. 'It's freaking me out that Sammy's with strangers and not me.'

'What about his father? Has someone been in touch with him?' There might not be a father on the scene. 'Or another family member?'

'The cops got hold of Carol's husband, and he's on his way in,' the paramedic answered.

'There you go,' Nikki said to Carol. 'Please try to relax and let the doctors and nurses look after you.' As Carol opened her mouth to reply, Nikki placed a hand on her arm. 'I know it's not easy, but everything possible is being done to make sure your son's all right.'

The woman slumped back onto the trolley. 'I'm sorry. It's so terrifying what happened.'

'I bet it was.' Even now, the moment when she was hit by a vehicle racing closer by the second when she leapt onto the road to save the little boy running from his mother was a vivid memory. Drawing a breath to quieten her mind on that subject, she looked around again, saw all but one patient being dealt with by doctors or nurses and the paramedics who were handing over responsibility for their patients. Jacqui was heading her way. 'Can you take this one, Jacqui? She's got a fractured tibia and other mild injuries, but is more worried about her young son who's being brought in by a policewoman.'

Jacqui was a doctor in her forties and very calm with distressed patients. 'The poor woman. I'm on to her.'

'Thanks.' Nikki crossed to the patient still without a doctor in attendance. 'Ash, what have we got?'

The ambulance officer looked up from the teenage girl. 'This is Katie, fifteen. Fractures in both legs caused by the bus running over her, dislocated right shoulder. She's been unconscious since we found her. Injury to the back of her scalp and a deep abrasion on the right cheek, where I understand she skidded across the tarmac.'

Nikki shuddered. It wasn't getting any better. 'She's the last of the serious cases?' Seven was what she'd been told when the 111 operator called, but she also knew the numbers could change once the scene was under control and panic had settled.

'Yes,' Ash said.

'Thank goodness for something. Bring her through to a cubicle. Georgie, you free?'

'Yes. Coming. '

'Good. Let's get Katie hooked up to oxygen and monitors so Ash can get on the road again.' To bring them someone else, hopefully not quite so badly injured.

Nikki began a thorough check of the teen, recalling the pain when the car slammed into her. Her hand automatically rubbed her thigh where it had been fractured.

'Want me here or with someone else?' Shaun appeared at the end of the bed. 'My patient's on his way to Theatre with the neurosurgeon and an orthopaedic specialist.'

'I could do with you here.'

Shaun had only started in the department on Monday, but so far he'd been impeccable. Confident and careful. Along with everyone else, she was glad to have him on the team, especially today with all the carnage around them. She wasn't thinking how attractive he was or what a distraction his steady blue gaze could be. 'From the little the paramedics know, Katie's been unconscious since being run over by the bus. Her legs bore the brunt of that, but the back of her head has a blunt force injury, and her face has deep abrasions.'

'Theatre's opening up more room as the few surgeries underway when the call came in are being finished and others have been postponed,' Shaun said as he read the monitor. 'I'll look at the head injury when you're ready to roll Katie onto her side.'

'Let's re-strap the shin so it doesn't move when we do that.' The bandage in place to hold the protruding tibia wasn't firm enough in her book. Creating more problems with the injury was not an option. 'We need splints on both legs.'

'I've got them.' Georgie handed her one and began to put the other on the opposite leg.

Shaun muttered, 'This cheek is open right through into the mouth. She's going to need a plastic surgeon after the others have done their work. It isn't as urgent, though sutures are required to help stem the bleeding. Plus we don't want her ending up with major scars on her face.'

Nikki huffed out a breath and gave him a wobbly smile. 'Welcome to Christchurch General.' It felt good working alongside Shaun. He made her feel comfortable about her efforts with their patients, even though she knew she was more than competent. It was only that sometimes her father's derogatory remarks throughout her life about her lack of ability to do anything properly sometimes made her pause and wonder if she could do better. *Not today, Dad. I know what I'm doing, and I'm doing it well.*

'You know how to put my skills to the test,' Shaun said with a wonky smile that had her looking at him twice. It was genuine and showed he wasn't afraid to admit his feelings, which was a surprise as so far he'd been a little remote with everyone apart from that smile. Could be part of the process of settling in to a new job, or today was catching up with him, as it was her. 'I've never been involved in a situation quite like this one.'

She had, in an Auckland ED a few years ago after a multiple car pile-up on the Southern Motorway. 'You don't appear too frazzled by it all.' He was handling the situation like the professional he was.

'I imagine that'll come later.' He was wiping away blood and bits of gravel from Katie's face so gently that Nikki got goose bumps. He was good.

Katie groaned.

Everyone stopped what they were doing and watched her. Her eyes opened, closed instantly. Another groan.

Nikki leant closer. 'Katie? Can you hear me? You're in hospital.'

Katie opened her eyes again, held them open for a few seconds. Closed them.

'She's coming round, and she's going to need

analgesics. The pain level will be high,' Shaun commented quietly.

'First I'll find out how long before one of the surgeons can see her, though I doubt there's a space in Theatre right now.' She had no idea how long it had been since the first patient had been taken into Theatre. Time meant nothing. Hopefully *all* the previous surgeries that were underway when this nightmare began had been completed. Picking up the phone, she looked around the department. Every single staff member was doing their utmost to help patients. Her heart swelled with pride. They were a good crew. Including the new doc on the block. Shaun Elliott had slid into place as though he'd been here for years and not just days. Yeah, he was a good dude.

Hours later—Nikki had no idea how many—the department quietened. She looked around and smiled tiredly. 'We're done? No more accident victims?' She should've known, but she'd been too involved with the young boy whose mother had been so stressed.

Turned out Sammy had fractures in his hand and elbow on one side, and had taken a slight knock to the head. Thankfully that had no repercussions. He'd returned from the plaster room and was sitting in a wheelchair beside his mum and dad, smiling at his cast where she and other staff had signed it.

'Not a one,' Shaun told her with a smile.

That smile tipped her off centre; it was wide and encouraging. Pulling on her straight face, she said, 'So we're done.' Except for all she knew, their shift mightn't be over, plus the waiting room would be overflowing with other patients requiring help. Glancing at her watch for the first time since all this started, she gasped. 'Three thirty-five. It feels later than that.'

'Time flies when you're having fun.' Shaun was still smiling.

How did he manage that when everyone else looked exhausted?

'Okay, everyone, the next shift is already seeing to the patients that were sidelined earlier.' Paul, the man in charge of ED, had stepped up beside Nikki. Wasn't he meant to be on leave this week? 'We've already seen to some of them. All of you get out of here while you can. But first, thank you for your dedication. You're amazing.'

The afternoon/evening staff began clapping, soon joined by some patients who'd been brought through from the waiting room.

Nikki squirmed. They'd only done what they always did, whether they had one patient with trauma injuries or numerous, putting everything they had into helping sick or injured people.

Shaun nudged her with his shoulder. 'Make the most of it. We don't get applauded often.'

Glancing at him, she gave in and smiled. They *had* done a great job. 'You're right.' Turning back to the room, she raised her voice. 'Thanks, everyone. Sorry to leave you with a heavy shift, but I'm ready for a shower and a hot coffee.'

Paul lifted his hand. 'Which has been catered for in the cafeteria. They've made sandwiches for you all. No showers there though.' He laughed. 'Go and unwind. And—' His countenance became serious. 'When you leave the hospital, go out one of the side doors. The media are all over the front entrance. If any of them ask you questions, you know not to answer them.'

A gentle reminder to keep their mouths shut. Nikki shivered. It could go badly when someone spoke up about a patient they'd dealt with after something as serious and public as this morning's bus accident would no doubt already be. After she'd saved Jordie in October last year, the media had hung out at the hospital in the quest for any information about her and the boy she'd snatched out of harm's way. Two reporters managed to get onto the ward she was in after surgery on her fractured hip, which infuriated her. She'd had little to say, preferring to keep her life private. Not that it was exciting enough for people to want to read about. Of course the reporters had had other ideas until a woman was murdered at a horse race meet two days later. Even then, she struggled not to regularly glance over her shoulder once she was back on her feet.

'Thanks, Paul. Come on, everyone. Let's change out of our grubby scrubs and go eat.' She'd prefer to go home for the shower her tired muscles were crying out for, but as head doctor on the shift, she would be there for the team.

As the day staff headed away to the changing rooms, Nikki lingered to go over some finer points with Paul, only to be told he had everything under control.

'I'm sure you have,' she agreed. 'I'm just finding it hard to switch off.'

'Perfectly normal,' said Shaun from behind her. 'One moment we're going non-stop crazy with desperate cases, and then suddenly there's nothing to do. I get it. I'm feeling the same. I suspect everyone is.'

Paul nodded. 'They will be. Go on, Nikki. Get out of here and start unwinding.'

'Yes, Boss.'

'Too right I am.' The man she'd known for years gave her a quick hug. 'You were amazing. And yes, I was keeping up to date with everything as I drove back from Nelson, where I'd gone for my grandmother's ninetieth birthday.'

'You're missing that?'

'I'm heading back up there tomorrow afternoon for the party. Stop dithering and go, will you?'

Shaun nudged her lightly, as he had earlier during the day. 'Sandwiches and coffee sound good.' His voice was low and gravelly, not something she'd noticed since he'd started working here at the beginning of the week. But then, she hadn't been quite so wound up before today either.

'All right. Give me five to put on some clean clothes.' She'd work hard at not racing outside and heading home. She'd rather deal with days like this one on her own at home, surrounded by the photos she took of birds and other wildlife. Photography had become her escape as a teenager when life got difficult facing new schools far too often. She had become very good at integrating herself with groups of popular girls, but the day always came when her father said they were moving. She'd have to cope with leaving her new friends, so out would come the camera she'd saved hard for. Far easier to rely on herself to get through whatever life threw her way. Her father had never given her or her brother, Ross, any attention or any of his precious time, and their mother had been too busy pleasing their dad to be bothered with her children. Thankfully she'd always had Ross at her side for understanding and the occasional hug. Then there'd been Brett, her husband and the love of her life, who turned out not to be the man she'd believed in but a piece of scum who had another woman on the side.

Life hurt at times, she thought as a yawn

gripped her. Yes, she was exhausted, but she wouldn't be the only one. Everyone had given their all for hours, and the toll was exhaustion. She wasn't thinking about her busy mind that would go on during the night, replaying everything. That was for later.

Shaun watched Nikki drag herself off to the women's changing room and smiled. Talk about a dynamo with patients. She hadn't stopped once, making sure all the victims of the bus encounter were being dealt with as well as looking out for the doctors and nurses as they too did everything within their ability to help the victims of a hideous accident.

Accident. The word reverberated around his head. The bus driver wouldn't have meant to mow down all those people. At least, Shaun hoped he hadn't. But was it an accident when the guy hadn't seen the light was red? He shuddered. Whatever the answer, the guilt would be colossal.

'You need to get to the cafeteria too,' Paul said.

'I know.'

'But you're wondering how you're going to get through the hours to come.'

He'd been deliberately avoiding that. 'Not quite. Though I'm sure it's not going to be a picnic.' He hadn't been on a picnic since he was a kid in shorts.

Paul nudged him. 'Follow Nikki's example.

She's one strong lady when the going gets tough.'
He'd been working with Paul when his life imploded four years ago, so the guy knew his history and understood how he struggled to cope with major incidents like today's. The good thing about today was they hadn't lost anyone. It had been touch and go with the man whose heart gave out for the third time, but Shaun'd been determined he wasn't going to die and gave everything he had to make sure of it. And he'd been successful.

If only he could've said that after his mate Liam's heart failed, but some things turn out to be impossible. Doing compressions when squashed into the tiny cabin of a Cessna plane five thousand feet above ground was one of those things. Throw in the fact he knew next to nothing about flying apart from the little Liam had taught him on previous flights, and it was the day from hell. Liam died before he'd had time to radio for help, so getting them down to the ground in one piece became his priority. At least he was able to keep the plane flying straight and steady until a flying instructor in the control tower talked him down, keeping him calm and focused until the wheels hit the grass runway. The plane bounced in the air, came down harder the next time and finally crashed. His guilt from that day was still with him, though quieter than it used to be.

'You still with me?' Paul asked.

Sort of. He'd been more than impressed with how Nikki handled the situation from the moment they first heard they were going to be overwhelmed with multiple seriously injured patients. The downside to having only one major public hospital in the city was needing to take all the cases, but Christchurch had faced some horrendous times before and came through well.

Likewise Nikki Marlow. He'd seen her on the news nearly a year ago when she'd raced onto a busy road to save a three-year-old boy who'd run in front of an approaching car. From all accounts, she'd been focused and determined then too, hadn't hesitated for even a second.

What he hadn't expected was to feel edgy around her. She made him look at her more than once. Many times more. Even in scrubs, it was obvious she had a stunning figure. Then there were those sapphire-blue eyes that seemed to see right inside him, which was the more unsettling of the things about her that got to him. He wasn't looking for a woman to become part of his life until he'd settled down in one place permanently. He was setting out to do that here on home turf with family nearby. In the meantime, he only did flings, and lately even those happened less often. He did want to find love one day, but not until he knew for certain he wouldn't move on yet again. Something he did every few months. A habit or still the past shaking him up, he wasn't sure, but he was now ready to do something about it.

'Coming, Shaun?' Nikki stood in front of him, a quizzical smile on that lovely mouth. She'd changed into fitted trousers and a floral blouse, looking so good it was difficult not to reach out and touch her.

Instead he concentrated on answering her. 'I'll be right behind you.' He hadn't ditched the scrubs yet.

'See you upstairs.' She headed away, leaving him to watch those shapely legs eat up the distance to the elevator.

Might be an idea to go home and put some space between them until his head quietened down. Except then he'd be letting down the team. When Paul announced there was food waiting for them, he'd sensed Nikki wasn't in a rush to join everyone either, but she was doing it. Therefore, so would he. It was important to be a part of the team, especially if at all possible this was to be a long-term job, not one that lasted only weeks or months. He'd made the decision to let go of the pain that had held him in limbo for so long. Shying away from something as simple as joining his colleagues for a quick—he hoped it'd be quick—get-together letting go of the day was not the way to begin. He would make this work. He would.

Five minutes later, dressed in jeans and an open-neck shirt, he headed to the cafeteria, where coffee and sandwiches waited. 'I'm starving,' he said as he took the chair beside Georgie after ordering a cappuccino.

'Given the way those sandwiches are disappearing, I think we all are.' Georgie nodded.

Opposite him, Nikki was chomping into one with a smile on her face.

'Good?' he asked.

'Delicious,' she agreed. 'Mind you, I could probably eat dog food roll right now and say the same.'

'Fried or cold?'

'Whichever.'

Leaning back, he looked around at everyone. They were a good bunch. Today had been his fourth day on the job, and he already felt comfortable. But that wasn't unusual. It was further into his time at a new job when he began to get itchy feet and started looking for other positions available in emergency departments across the country. New Zealand had a shortage of doctors at the moment, so he never had any difficulty getting a new job. Yet something about how everyone had worked together today had him feeling he belonged here more than anywhere else he'd been lately. Probably rushing things, he admitted. It was early days, and the hard ones were yet to come.

'Regretting coming to work here now?' Georgie asked through a tired smile.

'No, I was thinking the opposite. Today's been hell, yet I'm glad I was here to help those people.' He glanced across to Nikki and saw her nod.

'You fitted in so well,' she told him. 'It's as though you've worked here for a while.'

'Most EDs are the same. It's the people you work with who make the difference.' Something he hadn't acknowledged for a long time because to do so meant admitting he'd been lonely. After losing his mate, he wasn't in a hurry to make new friends. It wasn't fun being on his own all the time either, but here in Christchurch, he'd pick up with those he'd left behind.

'I think you're right.' Nikki sipped her coffee, suddenly looking a bit withdrawn.

Because she was head of shift and therefore had to remain a little removed from everyone? Or didn't she mix with people easily? Something to learn about her as time went on. He did want to know more about Nikki Marlow, which was unusual for him. He couldn't find it in himself to pretend he wasn't interested in her. Not that he understood why, and for some inexplicable reason, he didn't care. He was, and that was enough. 'I've worked in this ED before,' he said suddenly. 'I left three and a half years ago.'

Nikki's eyebrows rose. 'So you knew Paul when you applied this time?'

'Yes.'

'He never mentioned it.'

Knowing Paul, he'd have left it to him to decide what he told people about his past and why he'd left. At the time, he'd barely been coping with losing Liam and then breaking up with Amy, his wife, four months later. That had hurt more than losing Liam, and he'd carried some guilt over letting Amy down too. With the state he'd been in, he'd needed to get away from here before he made a horrendous mistake at work. He'd found having short-term contracts helped him get through the worst because he was always preparing to move on again. 'I imagine I did okay last time, so Paul saw no reason to mention it.'

Nikki's smile was wry. 'Fair enough.'

That was it? She wasn't digging for more info? Again he wondered if she'd been hurt in the past and kept things close to her chest. That could explain why she didn't pry into other people's lives.

'Damn and blast,' Nikki muttered half an hour later as she stepped through the door Shaun held open to go outside. 'I thought they were hanging out at the front.'

'They've probably seen others leave through the side door and figured you'd come this way too.'

A crowd of reporters stood around the side entrance, and their faces lit up with expectation when they saw Nikki.

'Dr Marlow, how many people died in the accident?'

'Nikki, did you work with the survivors?'

'Doctor, how serious are their injuries?'

Nikki balked, and colour drained from her face.

Shaun stepped up beside her. He wasn't leaving her on her own to deal with this lot. 'You know Dr Marlow can't answer any of those questions.'

Nikki gave him a quick look, surprise and possibly gratitude filling her eyes.

'Come on, we're allowed to know what the injuries are,' a woman at the front retorted. 'That's not revealing any secrets.'

Nikki stood tall and spoke coolly. 'I am not giving out any information about the patients we've seen today. It isn't right.'

As the journalists began shouting over each other to have their questions answered, others came flying around the side of the building, obviously suddenly aware someone of interest was here.

'Nikki, you know we find out everything in the end,' a male at the back called out. 'Like we did last time,' he added with a laugh.

She glared at the man. 'But you didn't learn anything important from me. The same goes for today.'

She was tough, though now resentment was taking over. He presumed last time had been when she'd saved the little boy. The media would've been all over the scene, and therefore Nikki. They were wolves, with no thought for the people they were chasing for info. Or the people whose details they wanted. He knew all too well about that after the death of his friend and how *he'd* had to land the plane with no real experience to fall back on. The media had had a field day as he hadn't been in any condition to deal with them. He hadn't forgiven them either. The pain over his loss and the fact he hadn't been able to save Liam had been huge, and it was like the reporters were rubbing salt into his wounds. At least they'd never learned that he'd lost his wife, Liam's sister, that day too.

It had taken a few months for their marriage to combust as they were both numb with grief, and he'd carried the extra weight of guilt. If he'd saved Liam, his friend wouldn't have missed out on so much living. No one ever blamed him for what happened—instead, they'd been grateful he'd survived—but that didn't stop the guilt. Amy struggled with her grief and how despondent he became. He'd struggled with having to face her every day, knowing her brother was gone. Finally they agreed to go their separate ways. Amy had found someone who made her happy again and had remarried last year, whereas he was still tottering from one place to another, looking for who knew what. Except this was the final move. He was stopping here, making a new life in old surroundings with family and friends nearby. Say it often enough and he'd come to believe it, right?

Shaun was suddenly aware he had been asked a question. 'Sorry, didn't hear what you asked,' he said to the crowd in general.

'Who are you? Another doctor? Or a friend of Dr Marlow's?'

Oh, great. 'I'm an emergency doctor.' Hopefully no one recognised him. He didn't need his past mentioned now. There was enough going on without that.

'Will you answer our questions? Who were the people who were injured? Were there any kids hurt?'

'I'm sorry, but I won't be telling you any details either. Now, if you'll excuse us, we've had a busy day and would like to get away from here.'

Voices rose as more questions were fired at them, but no one stopped them from leaving. Something to be grateful for, he supposed.

Until one man stepped in front of them, preventing them from going further. 'Do you know what Nikki Marlow did to save a young boy's life, Dr Elliott?'

Damn and blast. It'd been too much to expect to get away unrecognised. 'Yes, I do.'

'She's quite something, isn't she?' The man was ogling Nikki. 'Of course, you must be interested in her.'

Bile rose in Shaun's mouth. Punching the man's smug face would be too good for him. 'You obviously haven't a clue what you're talking about.'

'Excuse us, we need to get through.' Nikki had moved closer to him, not away. Tension tightened her face.

Totally agree. Shaun took Nikki's elbow and stepped towards the man. 'If you don't mind.' *Don't you dare mention the incident involving Liam and me.*

Just then, a photographer grabbed the man's arm. 'Leave them alone, will you? They're the good guys.'

Giving the photographer a quick nod of thanks, he kept moving with Nikki's elbow firmly in his grip. Her limp had become more obvious than usual. He'd read that her leg had been broken when the car hit her and noted she had a slight limp, but today being on her feet non-stop seemed to have taken a toll.

'Thanks, Shaun. That was creepy,' she acknowledged when they reached the sidewalk and were finally alone. 'Though I could've dealt to him.'

He bet she could've, but it was in his nature to protect women, especially one who intrigued him as much as this one was starting to. He'd noticed her the moment he first walked into the ED on Monday, tall with curves in all the right places. Not that she was the first woman he'd known to have a lovely figure, but there was something else about Nikki that teased him. He hadn't yet been able to put a finger on it. After today, he knew she was tough and kind all wrapped in one, there was a lot more that piqued his interest. 'I know, but I don't do standing aside when someone's behaving like that to a woman I respect. Or anyone else, come to that.'

She glanced at him, confusion overtaking the tension. Didn't she think he'd respect her? 'Still, thank you for sticking up for me.'

His eyebrows lifted. 'Why wouldn't I? You were amazing, the way you handled today's crisis in the ED. That has little to do with your doctoring skills, though they're top-level. It's about you as a person.' *Shut up, Shaun.* It was hard to stop yabbering on when Nikki looked so intriguing, thereby further ramping up his interest.

'Stop now or you'll embarrass me.'

Not used to compliments? Interesting. There was more to this woman than the doctor he worked with and the woman who leapt into traffic to grab a small boy as he ran amok on the road. 'Do you blush when you're embarrassed?'

Her eyes widened. 'Sometimes.' Then she spun around. 'I'll get going before any more reporters come looking for answers to their questions.'

'Did you drive to work?' He had no idea where she lived.

'I walked.'

'Then I'll give you a lift. My car's in the staff park.'

'Thanks, but the walk'll do me good.'

He doubted that with her limp, but he didn't argue. It was hard to accept this particular lady was walking away. 'See you tomorrow,' he called after her.

'Will do.' She waved over her shoulder as she strode away, eating up the metres like she was in a hurry to get away from him, the limp becoming even more pronounced.

Suddenly he laughed. What the heck had he been thinking? He and Nikki were doctors working alongside each other, nothing else. Besides, he was here long-term, not for a few months. He couldn't afford to upset his plan by letting Nikki in under his skin. When that had run its course, they'd still have to get along, and that could make working together awkward. *So turn around and stop watching her as she heads away.* Hauling air into his lungs, he did manage to turn away, not because he didn't want to watch her but because it could be interpreted as creepy, and he didn't do creepy.

He hadn't done long-term anything for years. Yet now he was setting out to do just that. He intended buying a home and maybe getting a dog, plus spending time with his family, with the idea of seeing how he coped. To get into a relationship with a woman and then find he couldn't do permanent would only lead to heartbreak. He'd struggled to settle anywhere after he lost Liam and then Amy, and knew he couldn't face losing someone else. At the same time, he was ready to give all he had to getting back on track with his life and maybe fulfilling those dreams of love and family he'd once had.

Spits of rain landed on his face. Would Nikki change her mind about accepting a lift home now?

He headed to his SUV feeling more optimistic. Only one way to find out.

CHAPTER TWO

NIKKI FOUGHT THE urge to turn back and accept Shaun's offer of a ride if he was still around. She was aching from head to toe after the crazy busy day, and the muscles in her right thigh where the femur had been fractured were tighter than normal. That would get worse before it came right. The sooner she got home and into a hot shower the better. On the other hand, she wasn't acknowledging the fact Shaun had a way about him that drew her in and made her want to know him better. He was an enigma she'd like to unravel, which wasn't something she'd felt when it came to men in a while.

But then she wasn't good at long-term relationships. Having to start over with new friends at all the schools she went to, she'd learned to be friendly while holding back a little. She did have two close friends from those years, and loved them for sticking by her throughout the turbulent times when she moved around so much. Other than Molly and Collette, and her brother, it seemed she wasn't made to be with someone forever, either a friend or lover. For her it all went back to her father and how he kept getting asked to leave a school because he bullied his pupils, demanding perfection. Her way of dealing with her father being the nasty teacher was to get onside with everyone else and be a great friend.

Then there was Brett. She'd fallen for him hard and fast, and he'd loved her back just as much, making her believe miracles did happen. She'd finally found the stability she'd wanted all her life. Their marriage had been wonderful, warm and happy. She'd no longer dreaded going home at the end of a busy day as she had with her parents, where her father was always waiting to put her down over something, or her case was on the bed waiting to be packed. Instead she'd gone home to throw her arms around the man she adored, and been hugged back just as strongly. Until she miscarried at fourteen weeks pregnant. That day changed everything. Brett wasn't there for her so often. She supported him through his grief but got little back, which was nothing like the man she believed she'd married. Then things got worse. One night he came home to tell her he was leaving and going to live with his girlfriend, who he'd been having an affair with for eight months. The woman was six months pregnant, and now that Nikki wasn't, he felt his loyalties lay elsewhere.

When she'd burst into tears and asked why he'd

had an affair, his answer was blunt and cruel. He didn't believe half of what she'd told him about her upbringing and thought she was a needy woman who no one could please. Look how she had behaved when she had lost their baby. As though she was the only one suffering. Well, he had been too, but he had another opportunity to have a family with someone else that he wasn't giving up.

It was clear he'd felt that if he stayed with her, chances were she might lose the next baby too, and that wasn't happening to him. Had she ever been right in believing he was so wonderful? Had she worn blinkers when it came to Brett, looking too hard for happiness? Or hadn't she been good enough for him all along? The worst was that he'd been so loving even in the midst of his affair. Moving past the hurt and disbelief had been impossible at first. If not for her brother and two best friends, she doubted she'd have got to where she was—comfortable with her lifestyle and finally beginning to wonder if there might be a man out there she could let into her heart.

Now Shaun was getting to her in unexpected ways. Working alongside him earlier, she'd felt his intense focus on the patient he was helping and thought he was wonderful. Whether it was the man with the serious head injury or the young girl with broken legs, he gave his all. He was thorough while taking the time to make sure the patient was taken care of, even when unconscious. Fast but careful. Surely a man like that would be the same with his family and friends?

He'd stood up for her when that reporter tried to harass her. The guy wouldn't have had a chance against her, but with Shaun telling him where to go, she'd felt truly protected and liked it. Too much.

A reporter had recognised Shaun. Why? What from? And when asked by a reporter if he knew what she'd done for Jordie, Shaun had answered in the affirmative.

Damned reporters. She hated them after being continually approached with questions about Jordie and her role in his life now. A few weeks after she'd snatched Jordie off the road, his parents asked her to be their son's surrogate aunt, making her weep with heartfelt joy, but when the media heard of it, it became a nightmare. Especially for the wee boy, as everyone wanted a part of the news and his life. In the end Nikki had told his mum and dad it might be best if she stepped back until everything quietened down. It eventually did, though when she'd met them for coffee and orange juice at a mall a couple of Saturday mornings ago, they were photographed by a reporter. Nothing major came of it, but it'd been a reminder they were still news when nothing else was going on.

Thunder blasted through the sky, followed by

a flash of lightning. Next Nikki was doused in heavy rain that looked close to becoming hail. 'Should've taken the offer of a ride,' she muttered under her breath. She was already nearly soaked through, and home was twenty minutes away.

Toot, toot.

'Ready to change your mind?' Shaun called from a black SUV that'd pulled onto the kerb in front of her.

She didn't answer, merely went to the passenger door and opened it to flop into the seat. 'I didn't see that coming.'

'Miles away thinking about your day?' Shaun nodded as he pulled back out onto the road.

'Something like that.' It wasn't a lie. Shaun had been part of the day.

'Where am I headed?'

'Fendalton.' She named the street where her small cottage was. 'Number five.' Then she wondered how well he knew the city. 'Do you need directions?'

'No. I grew up around here.'

'So you're a local.' She leaned back into the seat and rubbed her cheek, thinking how much more she'd like to know Shaun. The rain had cooled the air, and she shivered. Wet clothes didn't help.

'Want the heater on?'

'No, thanks.' They'd be at her place shortly. Then what? Did she invite Shaun in for another coffee out of politeness? Probably best to say thanks and head inside alone. They'd catch up tomorrow in the department. He was being helpful. Giving her a lift wasn't a date. A date? With Shaun? Where did that come from? She was obviously more exhausted than she'd realised.

He pulled into her drive and drove right up to the front door. 'Home sweet home.'

'It is.' She was proud of her house. Eighty years old, it had been well-looked-after by the previous owners, something she worked hard to keep up with.

'How long have you been here?' Shaun asked as he gazed through the window at the building, then her gardens.

'Nearly two years. I bought it when I moved back from Auckland.'

'So you've lived in Christchurch before? When you were growing up?'

'Only briefly.' Like all the places her family had moved to, it had been a short stop. Less than eighteen months for that one. 'Now I'm here to stay.'

'Family in the area?'

'My brother.' Her mother remained in Auckland when their father died and wasn't budging. With the past still hanging between the three of them, she and Ross had little contact with her, mainly brief phone calls for Christmas and birthdays. Mum wasn't interested in their lives, while she and Ross had moved on. She opened the door. No talking about herself. It wasn't something she did. 'Thank you for not driving off and leaving me to walk home.'

'I'd never do that.'

'Would you like another coffee?' The question spilled from her mouth.

'I should go home and get cleaned up.'

Should? Or would? 'I understand. I need to get out of these wet clothes and have a shower.'

'I'll make the coffee while you do that.' He was out of the car before she'd taken in what he'd said.

Shoving the door wider, she got out and slammed it shut. Now she was stuck with Shaun coming inside her house and sitting around drinking coffee. Perhaps she could stay under the shower until the water ran cold, by which time he'd have given up and left. Except then she'd be disappointed. She did like him. He was a puzzle, and she liked puzzles. No matter the source, they always had her trying to fathom the answers. Shaun certainly rattled her, even annoyed her, and then made her want to laugh and throw her arms around him—very odd. 'Come on. Let's get inside.' The rain was bucketing down. 'I hope it's not going to last too long.'

'This is lovely,' he said as he closed the front door behind them and glanced around. 'Did you do the decorating?'

Drops of water sprayed everywhere from her

hair when she shook her head. 'I wouldn't know where to start. The house came all done up, and I only changed the purple velvet curtains. I mean, purple velvet? Really?'

He grinned. 'I'm affronted.'

'Sure thing. They're your favourite style.'

His shudder was exaggerated. 'Might be all right for lining the dog kennel, I guess.'

'You have a dog?'

His smile slipped away. 'No, but I might get one now that I'm intending to buy a house and stay in Christchurch for a while.'

So he wasn't moving on like he'd done with previous positions? She'd heard from one of the doctors who knew him that he rarely stopped in one place for more than four months since something had happened that changed him forever. Something to do with why the reporter recognised him? She was yet to find out what that had been. 'With Christchurch being familiar territory, I'm guessing you've returned home for a while.'

'Being all over the place with different jobs, I missed my family.' He turned away to look around the lounge they'd entered on the way to the kitchen. 'This is nice.'

Okay, he didn't want to talk about himself. Something she understood. 'It gets a bit chilly in winter due to the lack of insulation in houses built so long ago, but I love it.'

'Show me where the coffee is and go take that

shower you mentioned, then put on some warm clothes. You're shivering.' So he wasn't one for dragging out a conversation for the sake of it.

'Through here.' In the ultra-modern kitchen installed by the previous owners, she showed him where everything he needed was, and once he'd assured her he could manage the coffee maker, she left him to it and went to get clean and warm.

If Shaun hadn't been here, she'd have stayed under the shower for ages washing away the day, but good manners won out. She was soon back in the kitchen, dressed in jeans and a sweatshirt and sniffing the coffee-scented air. 'Smells better than the cafeteria coffee.'

'I hope so.' Shaun was parked on a stool at the counter, holding a mug between both hands as though they were cold. He hadn't been drenched in the rain, but the house wasn't warm right now.

She switched on the wall heater and sank onto a stool at the other end of the counter, putting space between them. Couldn't have Shaun thinking she was interested in him other than as a doctor. Because she wasn't, right? 'You okay?'

'The day's catching up. It got a bit grim for a while. Kind of reminds me no one's invulnerable.'

Surprised he was admitting that, she agreed. 'True. Thankfully we didn't lose anyone.' Always a good outcome, though some of the patients were in for a long haul to get back on their feet.

'What do you do to move on from something like that?'

'Go walking in the hills.' Hiking was one of her loves, along with photography. Both helped divert her mind when she was overthinking horrific scenarios. 'In fact, I'm going walking with a friend on Mount Richardson on Saturday.'

'Perfect timing.'

'It is.' The weather was supposed to be fine and not too cold, though even if it turned out to be windy and chilly, she'd still keep the date. Right now she needed to get out there and let go of the tension brought on earlier. She knew from past experience she'd be on edge for days if she didn't do something physically challenging.

Shaun drained his coffee. 'I'm having another.' He wasn't asking.

'Go for it.' *Then leave me to get on with doing nothing.* She'd watch something trivial on TV or do a crossword or something else inane while trying to shove aside thoughts about the day, which included the man taking up space in her pristine kitchen. 'Another coffee addict, I see.'

'How else did we get through those night shifts without falling asleep when we were training?'

'True.' She pictured him sprawled over a bed on his back, out for the count, that broad chest rising and falling in a perfect rhythm. Why was Shaun Elliott taking over her mind like this? She wasn't immune to a hot man, but she rarely let them get to her. She wasn't letting Shaun, she realised. He was managing it all by himself. He'd piqued her interest while they were completely focused on seriously injured patients. That said a lot, because nothing, nobody, ever did that to her. Well, he could finish his next coffee and head away—get out of her house and out of her mind. He might be waking her up in ways she hadn't known in years, but she would not be following through. She'd learned the hard way how that ended, and she wasn't ever going to be put aside again. It had happened all her life by her parents and then Brett. Never again.

Her life was now about permanency, staying settled, keeping friends and not leaving town. She was done with moving from town to village to city, from one school to another, from meeting new people only to be hauled away somewhere else. She was in Christchurch to stay. If she ever found a man she could trust to love her for who she was and who didn't want to walk away when the going got tough, then she might take a chance on her heart, but for now she was happy as things were. Ross was here. Molly and Collette were here. She had the ideal job. A lovely home. What more could she want?

Her eyes shifted to Shaun. It would be wonderful to have a man at her side, one she loved beyond reason and who loved her equally. But was it going to happen? With a man she could rely on not to break her heart? There were no answers, and she wasn't about to make a fool of herself by finding out.

Her phone vibrated on the counter. Molly's name appeared on the screen. 'Sorry, I'd better take this.' Molly probably wanted to set up a time for going hiking on Saturday. 'Hey, how's your day been?'

'Pretty rubbish, if you really want to know. Which is why I'm calling. About Saturday. I can't make it. I'm sorry.'

Nikki felt her heart sink. She really needed to get out there and slog up and down a few hills. 'What's happened?'

'My sidekick quit. Right in the middle of a fraud investigation. I'm doing my best to fill in the gaps.' Molly was an accountant working for the police fraud squad.

'Fair enough. You do what you've got to do. I'll walk around Hagley Park fifty times.' Hiking alone in the hills was not a safe thing to do, even when there'd likely be others on the trail. *Likely* being the operative word. The tracks would be slippery after all the recent rain. If no one else was about and she fell and injured herself, she'd be in trouble in more ways than one. Putting her phone down, she got up to make another coffee. So much for getting out in the fresh air.

'What's up?'

For a moment, she'd forgotten Shaun was here. 'My friend can't make the walk.'

Looking thoughtful, Shaun took his mug to the sink, where he rinsed it out. Then he turned around and said, 'I'll go with you. I could do with stretching my legs.' He headed towards the front door before stopping and asking, 'What time?'

'Seven.'

'I'll pick you up then.'

She hadn't said she agreed to him coming. But it was too late. The front door snipped shut, and he was gone. She could run after him and say no, but she desperately wanted to get out in the hills and exert herself. Whether she wanted to do it with Shaun was another question. One she didn't have a definite answer to, and she wasn't going to waste time working it out.

Nikki didn't look pleased with him, Shaun thought as he drove away from her house. It had been a sudden decision to go hiking with her and if he'd taken the time to think about it, he wouldn't have run with the idea. But he had, and he wasn't going to regret it. It would be good to get out in the hills, and especially good doing it with Nikki. There was so much more to her than the exceptional doctor she was. Which was the case with most doctors, but for some reason he wasn't prepared to dig into, Nikki seemed to have more going for her than most. In his eyes, anyway.

The car surged forward as his foot pressed harder on the accelerator. 'Easy, man.' It'd been a reflex action to the thought that Nikki might be waking him up in ways he wasn't ready for. Returning to Christchurch to live long-term was a big enough deal to cope with without letting a woman into his life. A fling here or there was fine, but somehow he didn't think that would work with Nikki. She didn't appear to be your one-night-stand kind of girl. He wasn't ready for anyone else, not even this woman winding him up too easily. But he could do friendship. Walks in the hills. Maybe a coffee in town, even a meal together. Nothing deep and meaningful about that, just comfortable.

His fingers tapped the steering wheel. So he was going hiking on the weekend. Unless Nikki cancelled on him. It wouldn't surprise him after her stunned expression when he said he'd go with her. On the other hand, she hadn't instantly said no to the idea. Not that he'd given her much of a chance. After saying he'd pick her up, he'd got out of there fast.

They still had tomorrow working together in the department, which'd give her plenty of opportunity to say he wasn't welcome to join her. If she did, he'd be more than disappointed when he should be relieved. Coming home was hard enough. Taking on his first permanent position in more than three years was a challenge that he'd see through come hell or high water. The flat he was renting temporarily was pokey and cold, so he'd got on with looking at houses on the market in the two weeks before he started at the department. So far nothing had excited him. The most likely reason was that buying a home would tie him down when his instincts would soon be crying out to move on. Nothing new there.

He couldn't move again. The time had come when the past had to be laid to rest. Liam was gone. He was never coming home. He would not want Shaun to continue on the solitary road he'd started down the day he died. Slowly he was coming to see that for himself. He wanted a real life, not the lonely one he'd got used to.

Like other things in life, Liam's heart failure had come out of the blue. Or so he'd thought, until Liam's fiancée told him Liam had complained a couple of times about chest pain and done nothing about it despite her pleading with him to see a doctor. Since he was super fit, he hadn't believed there was anything seriously wrong. If he'd got wind of it, Shaun would've tied him to a bed until he'd been checked out. He still hadn't quite forgiven Liam for not mentioning the chest pain, but he was getting there. All part of letting go and starting afresh here.

Hopefully one day he'd find the life he used to believe was there for the taking. The one that included a family of his own, which meant the woman of his dreams. Amy had been that woman. They'd loved each other so much, but it hadn't been strong enough to see them through their grief and his guilt over not saving Liam despite knowing he wasn't at fault.

His phone rang.

'Hey, Mum, how's things?'

'I'm good. Heard the news and figured you were probably involved with those poor people hit by the bus. You must be exhausted, so drop whatever you're doing and come here. Dinner's on, and your father will be home shortly.' *Click.* She was gone.

'Thanks, Mum,' he said to the silent phone. She knew when to turn on the love, and neither she nor Dad would question him about what had happened to those people she mentioned. He'd be able to chill out and pretend nothing had been too hard at the department that day. Bring it on.

CHAPTER THREE

NIKKI DRAINED A glass of water as she swallowed pain meds before turning out the bedside lamp. Her thigh was giving her hell. Switching the light back on, she reached for her phone. Yep, the alarm was set. Off with the light. She stared up through the darkness towards the ceiling, desperate for sleep to push aside the chaos in her mind. Images of the teenage girl with her legs at impossible angles, the little boy who wanted his mum and his mum screaming to look after him and never mind her, tormented Nikki.

She concentrated on the breathing technique she'd learned when first working in an emergency department as she trained to qualify as an ED specialist. Low, slow breaths in through the nose, out through the mouth. Uncurling her fingers, closing her eyes, breathing slowly. She deliberately thought about Shaun. He made it easier than dealing with the other images forcing themselves into her mind.

When he started on Monday, they'd been busy

so she hadn't taken a lot of notice of him other than giving him details of who were the priorities, though his height and firm build had been obvious even then.

They'd worked together intermittently over the days since, and it was his deep, raspy laugh that had her turning her head to check him out when she wasn't focused on a patient. Sexy as all being, that laugh. But no, she wasn't interested in getting to know him beyond work. What about Saturday and going hiking with him? She'd deal with that tomorrow. Cancel the walk, find something else to do to fill in the day. *But* a walk was the best thing to do when she was uptight about work. Scenarios like today's reminded her how fragile life could be. She rolled over, pulled the pillow around her neck. She'd make a decision tomorrow. Shaun was a nice guy.

More than nice, Nikki. He's gorgeous.

Shaun sauntered across her mind as she drifted into sleep.

Blood and more blood. Broken bones. Screams. Pain. Nikki pressed her joined hands down hard on the man's chest, fighting to make his heart start. A monitor beeped. Another doctor held the pads as the current got up to speed. Someone shouted. A mother screamed, 'Jordie.' Car wheels screeched on the road. Nikki leapt off the footpath in front of the car. Snatched up the wee boy, held him tight against her chest. The car came straight at her. *Thud.* She flew through the air, still holding the boy. Banged down hard on her side. Pain overtook everything except the boy in her arms. Pain. Bleeding. More pain. Oblivion.

Nikki sat bolt upright, gripping the bedcover to her chest, panting hard. Sweat poured down her face, her neck, between her breasts. Her thigh ached, her elbow hurt. All part of the familiar nightmare, with more drama from the bus accident thrown in. When would they stop? Ten months since she'd rescued Jordie, and right now it felt like today.

After swinging her legs over the edge of the bed, she stood up slowly, fighting the shakiness threatening to undermine her stability. So much for being a strong woman who coped with anything. Being a doctor had its ups and downs. Helping people when they were ill or injured was what it was all about, but it wasn't always easy to put aside the images of pain and trauma.

A cup of tea would calm her. That and reading a chapter or two of the novel she'd begun the night before. Hopefully she'd finally get some dreamless sleep before the alarm went off. It usually worked, so fingers crossed. She could try thinking about Shaun to deflect other pictures filling her head, but he wasn't meant to be that important. His role in her life was as a doctor in the emergency department, and nothing more.

Except a hiking companion on Saturday.

No, not happening. She'd pull out of that in the morning.

'You looked whacked,' Shaun said as he crossed the parking lot towards Nikki first thing next day. 'Didn't get a lot of sleep?' There were dark shadows under her eyes, and the sparkly sapphire shade was dull. She was still limping badly.

'Not enough, that's for sure.'

'Is there such a thing?' The urge to reach out and hug her had him shoving his hands in his pockets as they headed for the hospital's main entrance. 'Should we go in the side door?'

'You're thinking about reporters? I'm presuming they're more interested in other staff now those patients are on the wards.'

'I hope you're right.' The way Nikki looked would have reporters making up reasons for why she appeared so shattered. 'Let's go for the side door anyway.' He took her elbow to underline his point, and was relieved when she went with him.

'What did you do last night?'

'Had dinner with the parents. They'd heard about the accident and knew where the injured people would've been taken, so Mum doubled the casserole and told me to get my backside around there.'

'She sounds lovely.' Was that longing in Nikki's voice?

'Even better, Mum and Dad know when not to ask questions about my day.'

Nikki glanced at him. 'You're so lucky. Most people want all the details even when they know you don't want to share.'

'True. Your family included?'

'My brother's a firefighter so totally gets why I hate talking about the bad days.'

Of course doctors weren't meant to talk about their patients, but there were times they needed to get things off their chest, and usually that was with someone they could trust to keep their mouth shut. 'If you want to go over anything from yesterday, I'm available.' No barriers between them when it came to work-related subjects.

Another glance came his way, this time with a frown. 'Thank you, but I'll be all right.'

'I'm sure you will, but it never hurts to share.' Not that he'd ever been good about sharing the pain he went through when Liam died, nor when Amy left. Nothing had been the same since.

'If only it was that easy.'

They were on the same page. 'Okay, we can share coffee and talk about the weather for tomorrow's hike. That way no one will get upset.' He was going for relaxed when he felt anything but. Nikki was lovely. He'd also seen a hint of vulnerability when she'd glanced at him. Before she'd pulled down the shutters.

'About tomorrow.' She paused. She would change her mind, cancel on him. It was there in her set mouth, in the now determined look in her tired eyes. Then she shook her head. 'Forget it.'

Despite what she'd told him, he'd bet Nikki hadn't slept a wink last night. 'Forgotten already.' He wasn't going to let her off the hook too easily. He wanted to go hiking with her, spend time away from here getting to know more about what made her tick.

Thankfully they'd reached the ED. Time to get changed into scrubs and find out what was happening in the department and put private conversation aside. 'It's quiet in here,' he noted.

'Long may that last,' Nikki gave him a small smile that inexplicably tugged at his heartstrings. 'I'm not asking for a slow day with nothing serious because that'd definitely tempt trouble, but I can hope for a quiet hour or two to start with.'

'I'm with you.' He swallowed. With her in more ways than he'd have believed possible given how he wasn't ready for a woman to come into his life. Went to show how Nikki had edged in under his skin with her calm, strong manner during yesterday's mayhem. She'd been professional as well as compassionate. Admirable and downright nice. Qualities that were important to him. *Not looking, eh?* He *was* remaining single for a long time yet.

There were other things he needed to concentrate on before contemplating looking for a woman to share his life with. Settling down permanently was top of that list. Having a woman in his life meant risking his heart. It didn't need a battering when it was only now recovering from his losses.

'Hello, you two,' Michaela called from the hub. 'Looks like you could do with a few more hours sleep.'

'Thanks, Doc,' Shaun quipped. 'How was your night?'

'Not too bad for a Thursday. The usual drunks with broken noses and twisted ankles, a cardiac arrest around midnight, an appendicitis, and so on. Nothing as horrific as yesterday.' Michaela stood up, stretching her back. 'We did have a reporter sneak in with a patient, hoping to get some answers to questions about the victims of the bus incident. Security dealt with him fast.'

Nikki shook her head. 'Seriously? He believed he'd learn something titillating at that time of the night?' The loathing was strong in her voice. 'Some reporters don't give a toss for the people they upset.' She'd know after saving that boy.

As did he from his experience of landing the Cessna with Liam aboard. 'They're not all bad, but some are loathsome.'

'Right. I'm getting changed,' Nikki said. 'Then having coffee before we get started.'

He watched her limp away, head high, back

straight as though no one should notice her un-
even walk. Those tight, light blue jeans emphasised her shapely legs and firm muscles. Nothing
like long legs to turn up the heat in his body. Was
Nikki still hiking tomorrow? She had to be in
pain to be walking like that. Was that why she'd
been going to cancel? If so, now he'd accept that
maybe she should.

'Her leg plays up whenever she spends too
much time on it,' Michaela commented matter-
of-factly.

'We never stopped yesterday, and I imagine
bending over beds doesn't help either.'

'Don't say a word if you want a peaceful day.'
Michaela grinned.

No surprise there. 'Got you.' Seemed Nikki
didn't go for sympathy. He presumed the limp
was a result of the injury where that car hit her.
There'd been mention of a fracture in some of
the articles about her grabbing the kid, but if he
wanted to find out more, he'd ask Nikki, no one
else. He headed for the men's changing room.
The thought of coffee to go with the egg roll he'd
bought on the way in was making him salivate.

Nikki swallowed coffee and light analgesics as
she watched Shaun decimate his egg roll. 'That
looks yummy.' Her apricot croissant was tasty,
but for some reason, his breakfast looked better.

Nothing to do with the long fingers that picked up the roll. Nothing at all.

'Wish I'd bought two,' he said as he screwed up the paper bag it came in. 'That's not a bad café over the road.'

'Suzie's?'

He nodded.

'Everyone's favourite. Most of the hospital staff go there.'

'So you drove today.'

'Can't trust the weather at the moment.' Her leg wasn't in the mood for striding out the kilometres from home, which was a concern if she didn't cancel tomorrow. Except she was desperate to get out in the hills. Walking with Shaun would be a bonus if she stopped thinking of reasons to avoid him. Maybe she wouldn't cancel on him. Sitting here, she felt a little wound up and warm. Even in shapeless scrubs, his body appeared sexy. There was a light stubble on his chin, which made her palms itch. He was too unsettling when she wasn't concentrating on anything else. Scary. It was so unlike her to get rattled around any man, good-looking or not. 'Anyway, I'm going shopping after work.' The new filter she'd ordered for her camera had arrived, and she wanted to use it tomorrow.

His smile said he knew she wasn't being totally honest, and that he didn't care. Kind of a new experience for her. 'From what I saw when

I looked up the forecast, today's meant to be fine all day,' he said.

So was tomorrow. She'd checked when looking for an excuse not to go hiking with him. Her leg would hurt like crazy until she warmed up, but her head would hurt worse if she didn't get out in the air and quieten down all the noise going on in there. Those were things she would not tell Shaun. She didn't do sharing personal concerns. The last thing she wanted was sympathy.

'Hey, mind if I join you?' Michaela sank onto a chair between them.

Michaela was the distraction she needed. 'Go for it.' No more taking sneak peeks at Shaun and wondering what lay behind his doctor façade.

'Want coffee?' the man filling her head asked Michaela.

'Love one.'

'Nikki, another?'

'Please.' His husky voice sent a shiver down her spine. She needed to get working and find something that required total concentration so she could put Shaun out of her head except when it came to patients. Easy to think, harder to make happen.

A couple of hours later, Shaun stood at the end of the counter where she was requesting an on-line prescription for a little girl with an infection in both ears. 'Can you take a look at my patient when you've got a moment, Nikki?'

'Sure. What's up?'

'Josie Lane, fifty-four, mild concussion after falling off a ladder, fractured ulna and radius, right side.'

Nikki looked up at Shaun. 'But?'

'You're on to it.' Concern filled his face. 'The wounds occurred three days ago. Her husband brought her into the department then. He was the one who filled in the triage nurse and follow-up doctor on what had happened.'

'Who saw her?'

'Jack. He's tagged her notes with a caution—says he wasn't sure if the husband was being truthful about a fall from a ladder or covering up some abuse. Not a lot he could do when Josie insisted on going home after her arm was put in a cast.'

'I hate these cases. My heart goes out to anyone who might be abused. The trouble is that we can't be certain that's what's happening unless the victim says so, and most times they refuse to do that.'

'For fear of more abuse once they leave here.' Shaun sat at the computer next to her and brought up Josie's notes. 'I'm going to get her arm X-rayed again to make sure it hasn't got worse. I've seen fresh bruises on her abdomen. She was quick to pull her top down when she realised I'd noticed them.'

'Is the husband with her?'

'He's gone to the pharmacy to collect the script I ordered. I told them to take their time so I could talk to you.'

'I'll see her now.' Nikki pushed up from her chair.

'Hopefully she might be a little more open speaking with a female doctor.'

Glad he'd noticed. Nikki bit down on her bottom lip to keep that to herself. 'I'll see what I can do. No promises.'

'Nikki? I get it. These cases are the most difficult when it comes to learning what truly happened. Cubicle ten,' he added.

She headed down the line of cubicles until she reached number ten. The woman looked on edge. 'Hello, Josie. I'm Dr Marlow. Call me Nikki. I hear you had a fall a few days ago.'

'Yes.' Her fingers were scratching at the bedcover. She lowered her head so as not to meet Nikki face-on.

'So what brings you back here today? Another fall?'

The woman was clothed from neck to feet. It must've been a fluke that her top rode up when Shaun was with her.

'Sort of. I slipped down the stairs during the night while going to the bathroom.' She was talking too fast, as though trying to get everything out of the way.

Nikki closed the curtains and nodded at Georgie standing on the other side of the bed. 'I think we should give you a full check over to make sure you haven't got any other serious injuries. Is that all right?'

'No. The other doctor checked my arm, said I need an X-ray again. I don't need anything else.'

'Did you bump your head this time?' Nikki carefully felt around Josie's skull.

'No.'

'It feels all right. Now can I check your tummy?' To see the bruises Shaun mentioned. It was an area often struck by an abusive partner because it could be kept hidden.

'Why?'

'I like to be thorough. Can't send you home without being certain there're no other injuries that need attention.'

Josie loosely wrapped her arms around her waist. 'I only came because my arm's still hurting. Nothing else is wrong.'

Nikki sat on the edge of the bed. 'Josie, did you truly fall off a ladder the other day?'

No reply.

'Do you want to tell me what happened?'

Blink, blink. Those fingers tightened.

'We can get you help. Also, we can prevent your husband from coming in here while you talk to someone.'

Josie swung her head back and forth vigorously. 'No.'

No surprise there. 'Have you talked to anyone about what's going on?'

'Nothing to tell.'

'Hey, mate, another doctor's with Josie. Come and wait here until she's finished.' By the sound of it, Shaun wasn't far away and was warning her the husband was back while trying to keep him away until she'd finished talking to Josie.

The curtain was flung aside. 'Hey, babe. I've got your meds. Let's get outta here.'

'Not so fast.' Shaun was right behind him. 'Josie's going to have her arm X-rayed before you go anywhere.'

'Nah, she's not. The arm's good. Just takes time for the pain to stop. Come on, babe.'

Josie was sliding off the bed to stand up, not looking at anybody. 'Okay.'

'Josie, you need another X-ray so we can tell if the bones are healing,' Nikki told her quietly. It wasn't usual to do that, but then, neither was an abusive relationship.

'I'm good to go.' This time the distressed woman looked Nikki right in the eye. 'Thanks for your help.'

She hadn't achieved a thing. Her stomach knotted. How she hated these cases. It would be easy to turn around and berate the smug-looking man reaching for Josie's other arm, but that'd only make matters worse for Josie. In the end, the decision to get help was Josie's. All Nikki could do was put it out there that help was available when she was ready, if she found the courage to follow through.

Nikki swallowed the bile in her mouth. Her father had abused her mother mentally non-stop. Ignoring her unless he wanted something *now*. Not coming home on time for dinner, then demanding a fresh meal, not what had been waiting in the oven. His temper was fast and furious and over in an instant, to be followed by ignoring everyone around him. He never struck out physically, but then, he hadn't needed to. His verbal bullying worked perfectly. He got whatever he wanted whenever he demanded it. Except at the schools where he taught. There they quickly lost patience and asked him to leave, and once more the family would be on the road as he searched for a new position. Growing up, Nikki and her brother had never lived anywhere, merely existed. Which was why they were both settled in Christchurch with no intention of moving away. Here was home. Christchurch was where they'd both made friends who'd stayed in touch from then on. It had been a no-brainer to come back when she broke up with Brett.

'That was a fail,' she muttered as she watched Josie drag herself away with her partner holding her hard against him.

'You tried. It's all we can do,' Shaun said beside her.

She flicked around. 'It's not enough.'

'I get that, but short of causing a scene, what else could you have done?'

Her shoulders slumped. 'Nothing.' It wasn't the first time she'd tried to help a woman in a violent relationship, and the result had always been the same. The woman did what her man told her. Just like her mother in her abusive relationship. 'At least being an emergency doctor, I do get to fix people physically.'

'That's not to be taken lightly.'

Nikki walked away before she said anything else. She'd already talked too much about how she felt. 'Who's next?' she asked the first nurse she saw.

Laurie smiled. 'A wee tot named Michelle. She's so cute.'

Nikki tried not to laugh. Laurie was enamoured with little girls now she was pregnant with one of her own. 'Why's Michelle here?'

The smile disappeared. 'She's got a peanut stuck in her ear.' Laurie leaned closer, said quietly, 'Why do parents leave dangerous items lying around?'

'I think you have a lot to learn about parenting, Laurie. From what I've seen in EDs, kids manage to find all sorts of things Mum and Dad think are out of reach. Which cubicle?'

'Two. Come on. I'm with you.'

When they walked into the small space, Shaun

was already there, talking softly to the little girl and at the same time calming a distraught woman, presumably the mother.

'Here's another doctor to make you better,' Shaun told Michelle. 'Say hello to Dr Nikki.' While he was talking, he was carefully examining the ear where the peanut must be.

'Oww.' Michelle jerked her head away. 'Hurt.'

Nikki sat on the bed beside her. 'Hello, Michelle. That's a pretty top you've got on. A pink elephant, is it?'

'Pretty.' Michelle nodded, earning Nikki a wry smile from Shaun.

'Oops. Keep your head still while Dr Shaun looks at your ear. I think pink must be your favourite colour. I like your pink trousers.'

'Everything's pink at the moment,' said her mother. 'Even your sheets, aren't they, sweetheart?'

'Yes, pink. Oww. Hurt again.' Michelle glared at Shaun, who had a pair of forceps in hand. He worked deftly to remove the object blocking the earhole.

'It won't hurt again. Here's the bad peanut, Michelle. Except it's a pink bead. Now your ear's going to be better.'

Michelle looked at the bead. 'I don't like it now.'

'What do you say to Dr Shaun?' her mother said.

'Thank you.'

'That's all right, Miss Pinky. Just don't go putting anything in your ears again, will you?'

'No. Naughty peanut.' She slapped at Shaun's hand.

Everyone laughed.

'I'll give you some antibiotic cream to rub in twice a day just in case she's scratched the skin,' Shaun told her mother as he grinned at his little patient with a look of something like yearning in his eyes. 'Otherwise you're good to go.'

Nikki understood that yearning. She mightn't be prepared to risk falling in love only to find the man was like her father or Brett, but it was her dream to become a mother. But to do that, she wanted a partner to be there for her child too, to be the loving dad she'd always dreamed of for herself.

'Nikki, the paramedics are bringing in a seventy-year-old woman with a probable fractured thigh,' Nurse Cameron called from the hub. 'They'll be here in five.'

'Put her in the trauma bay. What happened, do you know?'

'Slipped down the outside steps at home, apparently.'

'Okay, let me know when she's here.' Nikki headed to the hub feeling good despite worrying about Josie. Was that anything to do with Shaun? She couldn't see how. He did tickle her interest, but surely not to such an extent that she was waking up to possibilities about anything more than working together?

And going hiking tomorrow. Hmm. So much for cancelling. It wasn't too late. But something held her back, suggesting she should go for it and have a day out with a gorgeous man. Anything to blot out the nightmares she'd had last night.

'See you in the morning,' Shaun said as they left the department together at knock-off time.

'About that.' She paused, drew a breath. 'I'm looking forward to it.'

Shaun exhaled sharply. Knock him down, why didn't she? So much for thinking she was going to pull out of the walk. Instead she was looking forward to hitting the hills with him. 'Me too.'

He truly was. Nothing better than getting out in the fresh air and pushing his body hard. Could be even better doing so with a lovely woman who was definitely snagging his attention, whether she meant to or not. It was becoming impossible to ignore the warmth that enveloped him when around Nikki. She intrigued him with her smarts and her vulnerability.

'It wouldn't be much fun if you weren't,' she quipped.

'You think?'

'I can't stand gloomy people when I'm out doing what I love best. Can't stand them any time, in fact.'

'Hopefully I don't fit into that category.' Except when it came to sharing himself too much with a woman. Then he wasn't gloomy, more wary so not as much fun as he could be. Might have to put his fun hat on tomorrow to prove he wasn't too dull to be around. There was one thing he had to ask though. 'You're still limping quite a bit. Will your leg be all right?'

'It had better be. I'm going, no matter how it feels.'

'No surprise there.' He grinned, pleased with her reply. 'Seven still suit for pick-up?'

'Perfect.'

He was hoping for a perfect day in every way. Weather, the hike he hadn't done for a long time, and the company, though he already had no doubts that Nikki would be fun to be with. He enjoyed working with her, so why wouldn't hiking be the same? Sharing lunch on a hilltop as they took in the views beyond? His chest rose and fell a little too quickly. He was excited. Damn it.

CHAPTER FOUR

BANG ON SEVEN the next morning, there was a knock on her front door. Nikki shook her head. She'd overslept—something she never did—and now she was flapping around like a bee in a jar getting ready. Just as well she'd put everything she required into her backpack last night. 'Morning, Shaun. Come in. I'm having a coffee. Want one?'

'I never say no to coffee.'

'Even when we're meant to leave at seven?' she teased.

He smiled. 'I can take it with me.'

Her stomach knotted while her head felt light. That smile would do it for her every time. There hadn't been many in her life that could trip her up, but Shaun's did far too easily. 'Leaving five minutes later than planned won't change a thing.' The idea of sitting in the SUV beside him suddenly felt like it could get awkward if she fell into his smiles without thought. She wanted more, but receiving a Shaun smile was unlikely to change how she looked at life. She'd no doubt be in for a big disappointment if she didn't keep her sensible hat on.

'I take it you carry first-aid gear when you go hiking?' Shaun asked as he sipped the coffee she handed him.

'Of course.' Not only for herself but for anyone she might come across on the walk who needed medical attention. It had happened a couple of times in the past. Broken ankles on both occasions. 'Don't you?'

'Yes. I'm being careful, that's all.'

'I also carry an ELB.' Emergency locator beacons were the best piece of equipment any hiker could take when in the hills. Weather could change rapidly, causing people to become disorientated. Accidents also happened when least expected, and the best way to get help was to use the beacon.

'Me too.'

'Then we're well equipped if something goes wrong.' They could leave one of everything here, but somehow she doubted Shaun would. As the gear didn't add much weight to her pack, she wouldn't either. After draining her mug, she put it in the dishwasher. 'Let's go stretch our legs.'

'From what I remember of this walk, it will be more than a stretch.'

'How much hiking have you done recently?'

'Very little, but I do keep fit by running daily.'

Glancing down, she noted his trousers were like hers in that the bottom half of the legs could be unzipped to make the pants into shorts. If the day turned out warm, he might do that, and she'd get to ogle his muscles. Showed how boring her life had got if that was a turn-on. 'Do you mind stopping at a bakery on the way out of town? I haven't got any lunch.'

'Already on the agenda.'

'Cool.' Grabbing her camera from the hall table, she locked the door and followed Shaun to his vehicle.

'That's a serious camera,' he said as he started the SUV. 'Photography your go-to?'

'Totally. I'm in another world when I'm taking photos. It becomes me and whatever has my total focus. I'm into birds more than anything.'

'Glad I don't have wings.'

'You don't like having your photo taken?' She smirked. Then felt disappointed. It would've been good to get a snap of Dr Sexy. No, it wouldn't. That would be weird when she wasn't interested in him more than as a colleague—and a hiking partner. It also wouldn't be difficult to take the odd snap when he was concentrating on something else.

'Not fussed one way or the other.'

Maybe she could take a picture without getting growled at.

'Have you heard how our patients from the bus

incident are getting on?' Shaun asked as he drove away from her house.

A change of subject to keep her off the topic of photographs? She'd oblige for now. 'The four who were sent to ICU after surgery are still there. All except the man with head injuries are making progress. He had another operation late yesterday afternoon after a second brain haemorrhage.'

'Not good.' Shaun's hands tightened on the steering wheel. 'It freaks me out how someone can get up in the morning to go about their normal day only to have it turn to disaster through no fault of their own.'

Wow. That was quite a speech for this man. It was sounding more and more like something awful had happened to him in the past. Something that was behind his usual reticence to talk about himself? 'I admit I often feel the same. We see the repercussions from those situations, don't we?' After saving Jordie, she knew exactly what it felt like to have a normal day turned upside down through no fault of her own. It had been an instinctive reaction. If she'd hesitated to think about it then she'd have been too late. Would she do it again? Definitely.

'Yes, a lot of them. They don't go away easily either.' There was a new tightness in Shaun's voice.

She'd swear he *had* faced something horrific at some point of his life. As a consequence, had he lost someone close or been badly injured himself? Not her place to ask when they didn't know each other very well. Perhaps Shaun, like her, had learned to hold in pain and not share it with anyone. It didn't matter how often she'd been pulled out of one school to be dumped into another where she knew no one. She never got used to it. She learned not to complain. Otherwise her father would lecture her about how he was the money earner and she'd put up with whatever he chose to do. So when the man she'd believed to be the love of her life walked away after saying the *other* woman needed him more, she wondered if she'd ever be free of her doubts when it came to relationships. She trusted Ross and her closest friends, but she wasn't in a hurry to be too accepting of anyone else. Especially if it meant handing over her heart. Of course she was asking a lot of life, but that's how it was.

'Where have you gone?' Shaun asked.

'Nowhere important.' Not to him, anyway. 'Thanks for offering to drive. I'll fix you up for fuel.' He hadn't offered, just said he was picking her up, but she could play nice.

'That won't be necessary. I'm glad to be getting out and about after the week we've had.'

'Apart from Thursday, how are you finding working with us?' He might've taken up a permanent position and had talked about buying a house, but he was known to move around a lot.

Chances were he mightn't be in Christchurch that long. Something to remain wary about. She wasn't getting involved with a man who could pack his bags and move on without a thought for anyone else. Right, Dad? Brett?

'Can't complain.' He glanced across and smiled that devastating smile. 'You wouldn't listen.'

'Maybe not today.' Relaxing into the seat, she decided to drop any talk about work and go with the flow. Except with Shaun, that meant a lot of silence. He wasn't into talking for the sake of it any more than she was. She didn't mind. It was a comfortable silence, though the noise in her head built up as she thought about him. He was unlike most men she knew in that he didn't try to impress her, or show how wonderful he was, or talk for the sake of it. Yes, he was interesting—to the point she couldn't wait to arrive at their destination and get her boots on to hit the hills, so she'd have something else to focus on. He was quite a diversion when she wasn't looking for one.

He interrupted her thoughts. 'Where did you live in Christchurch as a child?'

'Halswell.' A rental property with no yard and little space inside. Her father wasn't into saving his teacher's salary, preferred to spend it on high-end motorcycles and showy clothes. The meagre wages her mother made working in shops went to feeding them. 'How about you?'

'Merivale. My parents are still there, though

they've handed over the gardening and upkeep of the property to experts. They're in their seventies and tell everyone their spare time's now for fun. The real reason is Mum was a very keen gardener, but arthritis prevents her from continuing, and she doesn't like the place looking in the least messy because it never did when she looked after it.'

Merivale was high-end, unlike Halswell. 'Your father's not interested.'

'No way. Gardens are for looking at, not for spending hours on your hands and knees, pulling weeds.'

'I agree with him. There's nothing like a well-designed garden to make me smile, but I'm no gardener. I tried but got frustrated when I put in plants and all looked good. Then they started growing, and the heights were all over the place, and nothing looked right.' That had been during the first year in her house. Since then she paid someone to maintain a simple garden while she stuck to mowing the lawns. 'What about you? Are you into gardens?'

'Never given it a go. Guess I'll find out when I get around to buying my own home.'

'Doesn't sound like you're in a hurry.'

'I'm looking, but so far nothing's appealed.'

She opened her mouth to ask more about him staying permanently, then noticed his hands tighten on the steering wheel again, and closed it. The last thing she wanted was to get offside with Shaun today. Instead she stared at the passing scenery and tried not to wonder what made him tick.

As if that was possible in the confined space. Every time she breathed in, she smelled spicy aftershave. Each time she shifted her head to the right, she noted firm trouser-covered thighs. It didn't matter what she did. She was totally aware of Shaun. Did that make her feel good? She winced. She wasn't sure. She hadn't done getting to know men well since Brett turned out to be a liar and so cruel. It was still hard to believe she hadn't sensed something was off in their relationship when he was having the affair. Her fault? Or his? She'd never really know, which made her wonder if she could ever trust a man to love her honestly. But it might be time to stop blaming herself for all that went wrong. It took two to make a happy couple, and Brett had been the one to play around. Not her.

'This the turn-off?' Shaun asked as he slowed down.

'Yes. You haven't been here?'

'Once a few years back, but I wasn't a hundred per cent certain I had it right. My mate and I used to do a bit of hiking when we had time.' Again his hands tightened on the steering wheel.

What was bothering him? He sometimes seemed to say things he instantly regretted. Odd.

Could be he was like her and not used to talking too much about himself to someone he didn't really know, so he struggled with saying things he didn't normally. 'There a problem?'

'No.'

Okay. 'Molly and I started hiking when I was specialising and she'd joined the fraud squad. We both needed to get away from unpleasant cases for a few hours as a reminder that life wasn't all bad.'

'We all need that at times, hence today.'

'Agreed.'

'So Molly's a cop?' He was good at abrupt changes in conversations.

'She studied to become an accountant and is now a detective investigating shady businesses. We and another friend shared a house when we were studying in Auckland. I said I was moving to Christchurch, and they came too. Molly's from around here. We were pals when I was here as a kid. As for Collette, she's from Auckland and couldn't wait to get away from there.'

'Too big?'

'Something like that.' An abusive boyfriend who followed her wherever she went in the city was the main reason.

'Not many people on the track at the moment,' Shaun commented as he parked on the grass near two vehicles at the beginning of the walk.

'Just how I prefer it.'

Shaun grinned. 'You wouldn't be a bit of a loner, by any chance?'

He didn't realise what he was asking. A loner? Or plain lonely? Both at times. Though not so much these days. 'I can be.' It was true. There were plenty of moments when the past came back to knock at her confidence and she'd withdraw from people, afraid of getting hurt again.

The grin disappeared. 'Why? You appear very outgoing, especially when you're telling reporters to go away.'

He was too shrewd for her liking. He'd have her spilling everything about her past if she wasn't careful. 'It's how I am.'

'And when you're helping patients, there's no holding you back.' This time his grin was gentle, as though he understood what she wasn't saying.

'You know how to win me over, don't you?' He could turn out to be too much if she wanted to remain a little aloof. The barriers were already crumbling, and she wasn't sure she could take whatever lay behind them, be it wonderful or bad, because mostly wonderful turned to bad anyway.

'I say it as I see it. Let's get our boots on and hit the dirt. I've been looking forward to this.'

'Me, too. And Shaun, I'm pleased you're here. I do prefer walking with someone else, and this will give us a chance to get to know each other better.' Did she want that? Yes, she did. What's more, she refused to regret it. She liked him a lot. She was coming to accept he might be on the same page as her when it came to getting to know someone more than as a colleague. Wary but interested.

'You talk too much, Nikki.' His grin was broad as he stuffed his foot into a boot.

'Smart alec.' She liked him teasing her. It made friendship real. Boots on and laced up, Nikki swung her day pack over her shoulders, her camera around her neck, and started for the track. Shaun was right behind her, making her more aware of him than ever. At least she'd put on fitted trousers that would flatter her behind. A laugh rolled over her tongue. Being concerned about how a man might see her physically was so unlike her it was funny.

'What's amusing you?'

'Nothing.'

'In other words, you're not sharing.'

'Damn right I'm not.' She laughed again and looked up at the clear sky. 'Looks like the weather's gotten over its wet mood and giving us a good day for a change.' She'd checked the forecast again when she got up and knew they weren't going to be rained off.

'Bet you came prepared for anything.'

'Not quite. I figured it's not likely to snow.' Not that it did out here. She concentrated on the track and setting her pace, hopefully one that suited Shaun. He appeared to be fit, so she figured he wouldn't want to dawdle, but he might think she was too slow for his liking.

Shaun followed Nikki, keeping space between them so she didn't feel crowded, something he sensed she might easily do. She hadn't denied she was a bit of a loner, though she hadn't come across as such with him except for that moment when he'd made the comment about being on her own. He had a feeling that, like him, she didn't get too close to many people, though probably not for the same reason. He had some great friends, but after Liam died, he kept them at a distance.

Amy had moved on and fallen in love with a decent guy she'd married in a quiet ceremony last year with only family and a few close friends, including him, attending. He suspected it was Amy's way of showing him he could move on too. He'd agreed that he should, but knowing it was time to leave the past behind was one thing. Making it happen was not so straightforward.

But now he had started. He was in Christchurch with his family and friends nearby. He'd got a permanent job for the first time in years. Though it was too early for him to be restless, that would happen, and he would deal with it. He'd make sure of it.

As he looked ahead, his mouth dried. Was Nikki going to be a step in the process? As in the woman who could make him happy again?

He stumbled, got his balance back to find Nikki had turned to see what was going on.

'Are you all right?' she asked, concern darkening her beautiful eyes.

'Absolutely. My mind wasn't on where I was going.' Actually, that's exactly where it was, just not on the track.

'Really?' Sounded like she didn't believe him.

'Really.' He wouldn't enlighten her about his thoughts. *He* needed enlightening first, and for the life of him, he had no idea where he and Nikki were headed. Except he liked her a lot. Anyway, what was wrong with having some fun and stepping out of his comfort zone along the way? It might help him settle into this new life he was determined to make work. 'Want me to go ahead?' He knew she wouldn't, but anything to get her turning away and moving on.

'If you want to.'

So he was hopeless at reading her. 'No, keep going. You set a good pace. I'm enjoying it.' What he was enjoying, he wasn't about to say. Those firm thighs in fitted khaki trousers were a sight to behold. So was Nikki's backside. Maybe he should've gone in front. 'How far to the top?' He couldn't remember the exact lay of the land.

'Roughly another hour and a half.'

They'd been walking around that long already. 'Not bad.' They were ahead of the time on the sign back at the beginning, but then, those signs usually gave a longer estimate so as not to send people on a walk they mightn't be able to manage safely in the suggested time frame.

Nikki paused, focused on a weka running along the track a couple of metres in front of them. Her camera was already in her hands as she waited patiently for the bird to stop. When it turned back, she focused the lens. 'They're not shy birds,' she said quietly.

No, they were cheeky and had no problem with strutting up to a person and taking a bite of their food if possible.

Click. Click. Click.

Nikki straightened. 'I am a bit OTT when it comes to taking photos, so expect the occasional delay if we come across something interesting.'

'No problem. What do you do with all the photos?'

'I had a calendar made last year using photos I'd taken of a variety of birds.'

'Did you sell the calendars?' Another side to Dr Marlow he hadn't known about. Along with just about everything else.

She smiled happily. 'I sold heaps of them. Couldn't quite believe it when the retailer rang to say she'd run out, and could I get another print run done ASAP.' The passion was gleaming in her eyes. 'It was great having my photos accepted by so many people.'

'Got any left?' It was over halfway through the year, but he'd like to have one.

She blinked. 'Yes, I still have a few. Do you want one?'

'You bet I do.' He meant it. He wasn't playing nice to get onside with Nikki.

'Remind me when you drop me off.'

He didn't believe for a moment that she'd forget. She was testing him to see if he truly wanted one or was only being polite. 'Will do,' he agreed.

Nikki started walking, her camera still in her hand, no doubt looking for another photo opportunity. There were always thrushes and blackbirds about, if nothing else. Though being cautious creatures, they wouldn't sit around waiting for Nikki to do her thing.

As they continued up the track, he thought about other times he'd gone hiking, mostly with Liam. They'd often done overnight trips and bunked down in a hut for the night, which he'd missed doing over the past years. Now he'd found someone else to do it with, someone he was getting on with. Hopefully Nikki might be open to other walks with him. Maybe even an overnight one at some point. *Don't go there.* That was getting a little intense even when lots of hikers did it. He wasn't ready to share a hut with Nikki, unless there were thirty other people there at the same time, and then it would be noisy with everyone talking and moving about, nothing like being in the bush with quiet surroundings to relax in.

'At last,' Nikki said when they crested the hill and began tugging her pack off.

Shaun stepped close and took it from her. 'There you go.'

She rolled her shoulders. 'That feels good.' Glugging at her water bottle, she looked out over the valley below. 'This is wonderful.'

'Not bad, is it? Wonder what everyone else is doing?'

'No sign of the people from those other vehicles,' she said.

'The track continues down the other side of the hill and around the bottom back to the beginning where we set out. It's a lot longer distance.'

'I haven't done it, and I don't think I want to today.'

'Good answer.' He wasn't keen to go much further. His legs were letting him know they were out of practice, and they still had to return to the car park.

Her eyes crinkled at the corners as she laughed. 'Thank goodness.' Opening her pack, she pulled out the chicken and salad rolls she'd bought at the bakery. 'Help yourself.'

'Thanks.' He dug out the berry muffins and cheese scones he hadn't been able to choose between. His plan to make a bacon and egg pie the other night had fizzled out.

'How often do you do walks like this?' he asked.

'About once a month, depending on what Molly's up to and my shifts.'

'Do you still lose any sleep over the accident where you saved that little boy?'

Nikki coughed, staring at him as though he'd asked the worst possible question. Then she rubbed her lips with the back of her hand and set down the roll. 'You think I lost sleep?'

'I can't imagine you didn't have at least the occasional nightmare.'

She nodded slowly. 'Did you know what happened before Thursday when those reporters spoke about it?'

'It did make the national news. More than once,' he added bluntly. Did she really think he wouldn't have recognised her after her face had been on TV and the news apps for days less than a year ago? Had she recognised him from four years back when he'd made the news for landing the Cessna in one piece? She hadn't given any indication that she had, but she wasn't always easy to read. 'When I got the job at Christchurch General, I asked if you still worked there.'

'Why?'

She'd intrigued him with her determination not to let the media make a big deal about her. Not everyone who'd done a heroic act wanted to avoid letting the world find out. 'I like to know who I'm working with.'

She didn't look convinced. 'What happened that day hasn't affected my work in any way.'

He hadn't said anything like that, but he let it go. 'What about your sleep?'

She shivered. 'Sometimes.'

'It's understandable. Did dealing with those victims of the bus incident bring everything back?'

'Yes.' She picked up the chicken roll again and took a bite. Her way of saying *no more questions*?

He understood, but for once he didn't feel like playing nice. He knew too well how those nightmares went, having had them screw with his life far too often. 'Have you seen anyone about the nightmares?'

'No. They're occurring less often, so I must be getting on top of them.' She shivered, which told him she wasn't being entirely honest.

He didn't push it any further. It was a long drive back to the city if he fell out with her. 'Those people who were injured in the bus incident will have their problems getting through what happened, and I'm not talking only about their physical injuries.'

'I can't see any of them rushing up to a pedestrian crossing any time soon. They were all lucky not to have been injured worse. Even the worst cases got through, though some have a long road to recovery ahead.'

'I agree.' Here they were sitting looking out over some stunning scenery, and they were back at Thursday's carnage. Not great. They were meant to be letting it go. He changed the subject. 'Have you walked the Milford Track?'

'No. It's on my bucket list, except these days you have to be quick when they open the site for bookings, and I figure it'll be crowded, so I'd rather do some other ones instead. What about you?'

'Did it a couple of years ago, and it was amazing, but even then it was busy. Like you, I prefer fewer people and more quiet. What about the Heaphy Track? That's another good one.'

'Molly and I did it last year and loved every moment. Each day the terrain was so different to the previous one. We started at the Collingwood end and came out at Karamea, where we spent a couple of days wandering around the area.' A soft sigh escaped her lips. 'It was whitebait season, so we made the most of that, eating fritters every night.'

'Can't beat a whitebait fritter. I tried whitebaiting as a kid but was too impatient to sit waiting to collect enough in the net to make it worthwhile.' He laughed. 'Far easier to pay a small fortune for some at the takeaway shop.'

Nikki returned his laugh. 'Not a patient man?'

'I've improved with age, though doubt I'd like whitebaiting any more these days than I did back then.'

'Take a good book with you and the time will fly by.'

'You think?' She might have a point.

'No idea.' She grinned and sent his stomach into a riot of need.

Standing up, Shaun downed half a bottle of water. Time to focus on walking and not the hot woman with him. 'Guess we'd better not hang around too long. There're some dark clouds on the horizon.' Not what had been forecast, but then, meteorologists weren't perfect. Though right now, he was almost grateful the forecast might be wrong as it was a good excuse to get going. This time he'd take the lead so he didn't have a view that had him thinking of sex.

Somehow he doubted it was going to be that easy to stop thinking about Nikki at all. She was gorgeous.

CHAPTER FIVE

NIKKI COULDN'T BELIEVE how relaxed she felt when Shaun pulled into her driveway hours later. 'It's been a great day.' She'd definitely sleep without interruptions from nightmares tonight. Despite them talking briefly about the horrors of Thursday, she was okay again, which was better than she'd hoped. Shaun had been quick to get them off the subject of work and onto more interesting topics. 'Would you like to come in for a drink of anything?'

He put the gear in Park and leaned back, regarding her with a softness he hadn't shown before. Nor was it what she was used to from a man she didn't know well. 'I've a better idea. How about we go for a meal later on?'

It was a lovely thought even though it meant something more personal than walking in the hills. Or did it? Was she overreacting to a simple invitation to have dinner together? Probably, but then, that's what she did. 'I'd like that. A lot,' she added without thought, and didn't regret it for a moment. It would be fun to go out with a man who had her heating up one moment, then cooling off the next as reality set in. Shaun was opening her eyes to a new world, and whatever the outcome, she was going to grab the moments they had together and make the most of whatever was on offer. Where the heck did that come from? Dinner was dinner, no more, no less. It could be a lot more. *Stop it. You've said yes, so make the most of it and see where this new friendship goes from here.*

Shaun was laughing softly, as though she'd made a joke. Maybe he'd read her mind. Not likely. She was good at keeping her thoughts to herself. 'What's funny?'

'I can't believe we're spending so much time together and how much I'm enjoying it.'

That was honest—if she could trust him. She had to. It was time to let go of some of her fears. He did seem to be thinking the same about their day. Somehow that made it easier to accept she was getting closer to him and more interested in who he was behind that sometimes withdrawn expression. 'So am I.' Opening the door, she reached for her pack. 'Where shall we go?'

'Leave that to me. I'll pick you up at seven if it suits.'

Plenty of time to soak in the bath and find the right outfit to wear, plus have a small wine for Dutch courage in case she suddenly got cold feet thinking of all the reasons she shouldn't be going out with Dr Elliott. Such as she worked with him, and he could make her happy, then walk away without a care in the world. Or he could turn out to be the one who got her back on track for the life she dreamed of. 'Perfect.'

'Anything you don't like to eat?'

'Very little.'

'Good. See you later.'

Nikki watched Shaun drive away with a growing warmth that was new. She hadn't felt excited about a date in so long. Strange considering she'd only met Shaun on Monday. Or was that how these things went? They'd worked well together, which had garnered a certain amount of respect and trust, and today's hike added to that. They got along like they'd known each other for months. Yes, he was waking her up in all sorts of ways. Usually that would make her hesitant about going out with him, but for once she didn't want to let the chance go by. She'd begun to feel she was ready to try to find love again, but every time she'd felt that since Brett left her, she'd got over it fast, not wanting to face heartache again. But if she didn't keep at it, then the future was already decided. A solitary one she wanted less and less by the day.

She wanted to love and be loved by a special man. She dreamed of having children to adore and watch over as they grew into adults and beyond. To share a home and time and holidays and problems. The only way to find that was to take risks and step out into the fray that was dating. Starting tonight.

Shaun smiled all the way home. He had a date with Nikki. He had to pinch himself to believe she'd agreed to go with him, though why he was surprised he had no idea. Only that Nikki was taking over his sane mind and turning it into mush whenever she came near. Of course he shouldn't have asked her out to dinner, but how could he not? She'd been sitting beside him all the way back to town, filling the air with the scent of the outdoors, reminding him what a great time they'd had and thinking how special she was.

Very special. Scary and exciting. He was home for good. It was exhilarating. He had to stick to his guns and not be sidetracked by memories of the fateful day that changed his life forever. His mate would've been the first person to tell him to grab whatever opportunities came along so his dreams became real. 'Yes, well, pal, I'm doing my best.' So far it was better than good. But he had to go slowly on the romance thing. That was the riskiest of everything he'd set out to achieve.

Where to go for dinner? Shaun pressed the call button for his brother on the car phone. 'Hey, Archie, where's a good place to go for dinner around here?'

'Depends what you're wanting. If you're trying to impress a woman, then I'd say the Blue House, but if it's a casual kind of night, then the Fish Box is ideal. They're both in Merivale.'

Not too far from home, or Nikki's place, for that matter. 'I'll check them out when I get home. How's your day been?'

'If you like watching seven-year-olds playing soccer, then great.'

'I'll come next week.' He'd been to his nephew Thomas's game the previous weekend and laughed the whole time. The kids were cute, running around after the ball, being very earnest as they attempted to kick it in the right direction. 'I've been hiking. It was good to get out in the hills and forget everything else for a while.'

'Go with anyone?'

'One of the doctors from work.' *And that's all I'm saying, because you'll have fun going on about me with a woman.*

'Not who you're going to dinner with, by any chance?'

Showed where his mind was. He hadn't given it any thought when he'd called Archie. 'One and the same,' he admitted. Since he'd returned home for good, he might as well involve his brother in some of what he was up to. 'Anyway, got to go. Thanks for those suggestions. Talk tomorrow.' He hit off and pulled away as the traffic light changed to green.

It was good being back among his family. They teased him about the itinerant lifestyle he'd been following, but deep down, they knew how much he'd been hurting. They'd supported him through his grief, and now he owed it to them to settle into a meaningful life. The life he'd once dreamed of and could have if he remained focused on now and not the past. Funny how his smile remained firmly in place. He *was* happy. What more could he want right now? Nothing. Everything felt good.

His phone pinged with an incoming text. At the next set of traffic lights, he glanced at it and groaned.

Don't forget condoms.

Brothers. Sometimes his was the best, and sometimes he was a pain in the butt.

Not bothering to reply, Shaun continued toward his flat, deliberately ignoring the pharmacy at the mall he passed. He didn't need to stock up on condoms. There were a couple in his wallet just in case. Anyway, he and Nikki were having dinner to finish off a great day as friends. Getting into bed together would only complicate things.

Unfortunately.

She was one hot lady. And interesting. He still knew very little about what made her tick, and wanted to know more before getting in too deep.

Hard to do when she wasn't very forthcoming about herself. Not that he could complain when he was reticent talking about his past. He didn't need Nikki feeling sorry for him. He'd done enough of that himself and was finally letting go, accepting the fact there'd been nothing he could've done that day to change the outcome. Sometimes life was a bitch.

Amy had moved on, showing it was possible. Now it was time he did.

When Nikki opened her door to him later, he admitted he might've started. 'You look beautiful,' he said around the lump in his throat. Yes, Nikki was attractive, but tonight in a sapphire-blue dress that barely reached her knees and showed a cleavage to dream about, she was something else. Her short black jacket emphasised the curve of her waist and tightened his groin when it was the last thing he needed right now. *Friends, remember.*

'Why, thank you.' She looked stunned as she stepped back, putting space between them. 'Want to come in?'

He shook his head. 'We might as well head to the restaurant.' It'd be easier to maintain control over his feelings when surrounded by other people.

'Then I'll grab my bag and be right with you.' She was gone.

Waiting on the doorstep, he drew steadying

breaths. That woman was not Dr Marlow. That was Nikki, the woman starting to wake him up in many ways. Too many? *Bring it on*, his mind retorted. He laughed.

'Share the joke,' Nikki said as she came out the door and closed it behind her.

Quick. Come up with something sensible. 'After our walk, I'm feeling more energetic than I have in a while. Thought I'd be complaining of muscles aching in places I didn't know I had any.'

'It's the fresh air getting to you.' She grinned over her shoulder as she got into the SUV. 'You need to get outside more often.'

That wouldn't be difficult if Nikki was happy to go on other hikes with him. As he backed out of her drive, he asked, 'Have you done any of the walks around Governors Bay?'

'Most of them. Thinking you'd like to give some a go?'

'I'm keen to. Today reminded me why I used to like hiking.'

'Strange how we sometimes stop doing something we enjoy, isn't it?'

Was she asking why he'd stopped? If so, he wasn't telling her his story, but he could open up a little. Somehow he didn't think Nikki was the type to start digging for more info so she could say she knew more about him. 'I used to hike with my best mate. He died a few years ago, and I sort of drifted away from doing it.' He'd gone once with some other friends, but it wasn't the same, like something was missing. Which it was, only it wasn't some*thing*, it was Liam. Another reminder of what had happened. Yet today he hadn't once felt that way.

'I'm sorry to hear that. I'm glad you came. I needed to get out there, and I won't go alone on long walks. If it helped you find your mojo for hiking again, then that's a bonus.'

'You're right, it is.' He hadn't hesitated to suggest he'd go with her when her friend pulled out, which said more about how comfortable he felt around Nikki than anything else. The fact she didn't delve into why his friend had died added to that. It was usually the first question people asked when they heard Liam was killed. 'Anytime you want to go hiking and your friend isn't available, give me a call.'

Her smile was open and friendly. 'Can do.'

See, as easy as that. Caution had taken a back seat, making him happier. Life was looking better by the day. Seemed he was already making serious changes, though getting close to a wonderful woman wasn't on the list. That wasn't because he wanted to remain single forever, but more because he was still afraid of falling for someone and then losing her as he had Amy. For a man who used to take risks about most things, he really had become a hermit when it came to sharing his heart. Now there was a lightness in his chest he hadn't known in a long time. *Bring it on.*

Nikki placed her fork on the empty dessert plate and leaned back in the chair. 'That was delicious.' Almost as yummy as the sight before her.

The dark blue shirt Shaun wore matched his eyes perfectly, drawing her gaze to the vee pointing down his chest. His blond hair fell in light waves over the back of his neck, and her fingers itched to run through it, to feel the silkiness. It had been a while since she'd wanted to be intimate with a man, yet it hadn't taken much to feel that way about Shaun. He was a hunk. Kind and generous to go with that. Serious when he had to be, light-hearted when he didn't. Not that he talked much about himself, something she normally didn't mind, but she longed to learn more. She mightn't be willing to hand over her heart, but she could have fun while getting to know Shaun.

He put down his spoon. 'I agree.'

If he knew what else she'd been thinking, he probably wouldn't. 'I didn't know about this restaurant. I'm coming again.' Who with? She shrugged. She wasn't going to worry about that right now.

'Something else you can give me a call about.' Shaun grinned.

'You're on,' she said without thinking. But

then, why not? They'd got on well throughout the day and over a wonderful dinner. She was realising how much she'd missed having someone in her life to do the things she enjoyed with. Not since Brett had she been overly keen on a man, and now Shaun was knocking at her door far too easily. Was he someone she could trust not to hurt her? Brett had been the opposite to her father, not aloof or selfish in the least. Or so she'd thought until the day he told her he was leaving her for the pregnant woman he'd been in a relationship with on the side. Call her a fool, but she doubted Shaun was the type to go behind his partner's back and have an affair. Not that she knew why she thought so, only that he came across as sincere about everything he did. He didn't talk a lot about himself and try to impress her with things he'd done. Quite the opposite. Of course, she could be wrong. Brett hadn't appeared to be a liar or selfish either. The problem was that if she wanted to find love, then she had to start trusting men more often. Maybe this one.

'I'm going to have to give you my number, aren't I?' He was still grinning. Another surprise, because he didn't do that often.

'That'd save me looking it up at work.' She grinned back. This was getting silly. They were like teenagers on their first date. Well, it was their first date. 'Time to go?'

'Unless you'd like a nightcap?'

'No, thanks. It'd keep me awake half the night.' She suspected images of Shaun were going to do that anyway.

Shaun stood up. 'Thanks for a good time. It's been a while since I had such a lovely evening.'

He didn't date? Come on. He was good-looking and hot. There must be a queue of women wanting to go out with him. 'You're out of practice?'

His laugh made her skin tingle. 'No, but it's not often I enjoy myself so much.'

She blinked. Seriously? Shaun said that? She'd take it as a compliment. 'Maybe there are some good things to come from that bus incident.'

'Could be. It struck us both hard, and now we're working on getting over it.' He pulled his wallet from his jacket pocket. 'Together.'

She was lost for words. For a man who rarely said anything personal, he seemed to be getting carried away. Not what she'd expected, but she liked it. The trust barrier was not going up tonight. She would continue having fun until he dropped her off at home. Unless— She swallowed hard. Unless nothing. Their day together was about to finish. Nothing else was happening. So why was disappointment filling her? Life was too short for procrastination. Look at those people they'd helped in ED on Thursday. When they left home that morning, not one of them knew how their life would change so abruptly. She knew what it was like to have everything change without warning—from losing her baby and Brett to leaping in front of a moving car.

Yet it felt like the time had come to let go and take some risks.

When he pulled up at Nikki's, Shaun turned off the motor and turned to face her. 'Thanks for an awesome day. Like I said, I've really enjoyed it.'

'You and me both.'

Hauling her into his arms and kissing her blind might not go down well, but it was hard not to. Nikki was temptation on amazing legs. Shoving his door wide, he got out before he made an idiot of himself. They had to work together, and if she wasn't on the same page, life in the department would be hell.

But it was impossible to ignore the longing for someone special in his life. If he didn't ignore it, he had to start taking chances on *everything*, and put the brake on thinking about how abruptly things could change without any input from himself. Thursday had been a shocking reminder of that, which was a good reason not to follow through on the longing heating his body right now.

Opening the passenger door, he offered Nikki his hand to help her out of the car. She took it, and he kept it there as they walked up to her front door, momentarily savouring her warmth through the sleeve of her jacket, pretending the need Nikki created within him wasn't real. So much for friendship. He had to be careful. He didn't think getting too close to Nikki could end comfortably. If they started something intimate, then he suspected he might not want it to end, and he wasn't ready for that.

Opening her door, Nikki turned to him. 'I haven't had such a good time in ages.' Her eyes widened as she watched him. 'It's true.'

'Nor have I,' he said softly, forgetting the warnings he'd given himself. His hand was on her arm, and he was reluctant to pull away. He could feel her muscles tighten, then soften.

Then she was leaning close, her scent teasing him, her breath whispering across the skin on his neck. Her lips brushed across his so lightly it felt like a feather. But it wasn't. It was Nikki, her lips, her mouth, her body suddenly pressing up against his.

His arms were around her, pulling her nearer so he could feel her breasts against his chest, her firm thighs meeting his. Opening his mouth, he covered her tantalising lips, tasted her, felt her heat, wanted more. Pulling his head back, he looked into her gaze. 'Nikki?'

Her nod was abrupt as she tugged him inside and slammed the door shut behind them. Then her arms were around his neck, and his mouth again covered by hers. Warmth filled him, hunger and longing following fast. Nikki was beyond wonderful. Deepening his kiss, he drank in her taste and her heat. So much for behaving. It was impossible.

His hands found her buttocks and gripped them, pulling her up against his arousal.

Nikki groaned, long and low, driving him crazy with need. Pulling back, he looked at her. 'Nikki? Are you sure?'

Her eyes widened, and those luscious lips curved upward. 'Oh, yes.' Then she grabbed his shoulders and lifted her legs up around his waist. 'Oh, yes.'

He was throbbing with need, and when he touched her heat, he found the same reaction. Wet, hot, wanting. His fingers rubbed her. She bucked against him. This would be over before they started if they didn't slow down.

'Shaun, please. Take me.'

He was more than happy to oblige.

'One moment. I need to remove my trousers *and* find my wallet to get a condom.'

Nikki slid to the floor and waited impatiently until he'd removed his pants, then reached for him, leaning down and licking him.

'Nikki, please. I won't be able to wait if you do that.'

She snatched the condom from his fingers and tore the packet open.

Her face lit up. 'Good.'

Placing his hand under her chin, he held her still. 'No, we do this together.'

'I intend to.' Her eyes were wide with heat and a need identical to his.

He took the condom from her and deftly slid it over his throbbing erection. Lifting her back up into his arms, he turned so she was against the wall. When her legs went around his waist, he touched her centre, moving back and forward until she cried out, and then he dived into that heat. Then pulled back to repeat the move, again and again.

Nikki cried out. Louder this time as she tightened around him. He let go all restraint and dove in as deep as possible, feeling her enclose him, suck his need into hers.

How long he stood there, Nikki's legs still tight around him, he hadn't a clue, but eventually she moved, and he lowered her to stand in front of him. Her face was pink, her eyes filled with passion, and her exquisite mouth tilted into a soft smile. 'Wow.'

Leaning in, he brushed a kiss over her swollen lips. 'Yes, wow.'

She took his hand and led him to a bedroom. Hers, he presumed since the furnishings were blue and pink. More importantly, the bed was large. And soft and cosy when they lay under the covers, their clothes on the floor, and Nikki's legs wound around his.

Placing a kiss on her forehead, he sighed. 'So much for dropping you off and heading home.'

She tensed. 'You're regretting this?'

'No, I am not.' He should have been, but he wasn't going there when he felt happy beyond reason. 'That was amazing.'

The tension left Nikki as quickly as it had come. 'Good, because we're not finished yet.'

He'd barely got his breath back, but so what? Reaching for Nikki, he rose above her and set out to discover every inch of her beautiful body. Kissing and touching warm velvety skin from her face to her toes and everything in between, he couldn't stop. She was wonderful.

Nikki's hands were on his back, his thighs, his chest, his erection, heating him throughout. Turning him on as fast as the first time. He reached for his wallet, glad for a second condom or this wouldn't be happening.

'Let me.' The foil packet was gone, and Nikki was dealing with the condom.

Then he was being covered.

Taking Nikki in his hands, he slid her beneath him and gazed into her eyes, falling into her warmth and heat and sex. Knowing nothing but this. Being intimate with Nikki. Giving her more of himself than he'd thought possible.

CHAPTER SIX

'WHAT HAVE I DONE?' Nikki groaned the next morning as she rolled over in the twisted sheets.

Shaun had left a short while after they'd made love for the second time. She'd been tucked up beside him, savouring the moment with him, his hand rubbing light circles on her back. She'd known it wasn't forever but had been happy with what she got. When he hauled himself out of bed and shrugged into his clothes, she'd wanted to beg him to stay longer but instead enjoyed the view for the brief moments before he was fully dressed.

He'd leaned down to kiss her cheek. 'Again, thank you for an amazing day.'

'And night,' she'd whispered.

He'd nodded. 'You're right there. But I think I'd better be going so we don't overdo things and live to regret it in the daylight.'

He was right even though she hated to admit it. 'I agree.'

'Bye.' Then he was gone.

She'd got up to check the door was locked behind him before crawling back into bed filled with wonder and a deep longing for more of what they'd shared all day and night.

She'd been getting ahead of herself. They'd barely met and she was thinking of the future. So unlike her. Usually her way was to think more about the person than the effects he had on her. But then she hadn't had such intense desire for a man since Brett and had believed it might never happen again.

Rolling over, she'd tucked the covers up around her neck to keep warm, believing she'd lie awake most of what was left of the night.

Got that wrong, hadn't she? She couldn't remember much at all after that. Now she was wide awake, she wasn't feeling quite so relaxed about having made out with Shaun. Not once but twice, and she'd been the instigator, kissing him when he was about to leave. Not that he'd been far behind her when it came to getting turned on and ready for sex.

But reality was kicking in. They were workmates who'd spent a day together hiking and enjoying a meal. That should've been it. Friends, not lovers.

But they'd had sex. Twice. Mind-blowing sex that she wasn't going to forget in a hurry. He was good. Sexy and hot, and very satisfying. It wouldn't be easy to forget how good whenever she saw him and that would be often in the ED when rostered on the same shift. He'd been right to go when he did, but part of her regretted it. They'd been great together.

She had to focus on the fact Shaun had a history of taking short-term positions and that while his current one was supposedly permanent, the odds were stacked against him staying for long. He'd said something about buying a house and maybe getting a dog, but had he seriously started along that track, or had he been a bit casual about the houses he'd looked at? He'd mentioned doing more walks with her, but how long would he stay here? After her childhood spent regularly moving from place to place, she intended staying put. Even if she fell in love with a man who had other ideas about where he wanted to live permanently. That was the word that mattered to her. *Permanently.* At the moment, she didn't think Shaun was capable of that.

She had no idea where that thought came from. It was too soon for her to ask him if he was serious about settling down. Whatever the circumstances of his friend's death, they might be behind his inability to have settled so far. If only he'd share a bit more with her. Of course she was out of line, considering she didn't like talking about Brett and how he'd left her for the other woman, leaving her feeling unworthy and wary of taking a risk, of being hurt again.

Her phone rang. Molly. Not in the mood to talk

about Shaun to her friend, who would ask about the hike, she ignored it.

Everyone needed a best buddy to share certain things with, but not when she was still working through her feelings about having slept with Shaun.

Nikki didn't want to be cautious whenever she saw him, but she knew so little about him. Believing she could trust him not to hurt her was all very well. Been there, done that. But if she loosened up, maybe she could have it all. Greedy? Why not? Other people had it all. Maybe it was her turn.

Her phone rang again. No doubt Molly trying again. But no, it was Ross.

'Hey, Nikki, got anything planned for today?'

'Not a thing.' She wasn't calling Shaun to see if he'd like to go for another walk. That would appear too eager. She was going to take things quietly—for today anyway. That was kind of what they'd agreed on when he left last night.

'Good. Haul on some warm clothes and meet us at Hagley Park. Logan wants to see Auntie Nikki and go for burgers and chips afterwards.'

'Catch you shortly.' Excellent. Something to keep her mind busy so she couldn't keep rerunning last night and that amazing sex. She was starting to see there couldn't be a repeat. It just wouldn't work. They couldn't have a relationship while working together.

Other staff did.

It could get awkward if something went wrong between them. Looking for trouble? Or looking out for her heart? Last night she was willing to take a risk. Not so much this morning. Reality was a wake-up call. Chances were Shaun wouldn't want to be obvious about their day out around other staff members either. He might've thought about what they'd done and decided it wasn't for him. One night was enough. Was that the real reason he'd left? Even knowing it had probably been for the best, she hoped not. She was coming up with so many reasons it was doing her head in.

This was ridiculous. She leapt out of bed and went to turn on the coffee machine before showering away the scents of last night and giving her hair a good wash. Time to get out and about, and stop overthinking everything. That only spoilt those amazing memories, which was the last thing she wanted right now. She really didn't know if she was coming or going with this so-called relationship.

On Monday morning, Nikki walked into the ED feeling uncomfortable. Would Shaun be okay around her? She worried he'd have been busy overthinking everything too and would want nothing more to do with her. That'd be awkward around the other staff.

'Morning, Nikki. How was your weekend?' Paul asked.

'Great. Went for a hike on Saturday, gave the muscles a good stretch. What about you?'

'We went up to Kaikoura for a friend's birthday and stayed the night.'

'It's a lovely spot for a break, isn't it?'

'Sure is. Right, let me run through what's going on before I head home for a shower and sleep.'

'It seems quite busy for this early on a Monday morning,' Shaun said from behind Nikki.

The clock read six forty. 'Can't always predict what's going to happen.'

Shaun gave her an open smile. 'I know, but no harm in wishing for a quiet start.'

The worry rattling in her chest subsided. He didn't appear to have any problems about their weekend. 'Right, let's get this underway.'

Other staff were beginning to appear, and soon everyone was listening to Paul's summary of patients and what had been arranged about treatment.

The bell at the ambulance bay rang loudly, cutting through the discussion going on.

'That'll be the woman involved in a car accident at Hillmorton,' Paul said.

'I'll take it.' Shaun looked to Nikki for agreement.

'All yours. Georgie, go with him.' Sipping coffee, Nikki concentrated on allocating patients to everyone else. No such thing as too much caffeine early in the morning. Especially this morning after tossing and turning for hours before finally dropping into a restless sleep around midnight. Shaun had been in her head all the time. Could they have a relationship or a long fling, or should they quit while they were ahead so neither of them got hurt?

'Morning, Nikki. I hear there's a girl needing an appendectomy waiting for me.'

She glanced up at Jack. 'Cubicle one. Jenny Brown. Fourteen.' She'd just finished reading the notes on screen. 'Have a good weekend?'

'I was on call. It was busy. You?'

'No complaints.' The phone was ringing. 'I'll be with you in a minute.' Picking up the phone she said, 'Emergency Department, Dr Marlow speaking.'

'Morning, Nikki. It's Darren. Can you send your patient up to Radiology now? We're all set to take his X-rays.' *Click.* The man was gone.

Nikki shrugged. She was used to Darren's abrupt manner. Pressing the number for the orderlies, she arranged for one to come along right away.

A trolley pushed by paramedics came past with Shaun walking at the side, watching the woman lying on top. 'Meredith, can you hear me?'

She groaned.

'You're in the hospital emergency department. I'm Shaun, a doctor.'

Another groan.

Nikki got up to follow in case she was needed.

'The paramedics think you banged your head on the steering wheel. Do you know if that's right?'

The woman dipped her head slightly.

'We need Radiology on alert. Right arm's fractured. Internal swelling in the lower abdomen.' Shaun flicked Nikki a glance. 'She wasn't wearing her seat belt.'

Grand. When would people learn not to takes risks behind the wheel? 'What did she impact into?'

'Power pole,' one of the paramedics answered. 'She ended up twisted around the steering wheel and half in the foot bay. According to a bystander, she was unconscious for about ten minutes.'

'Want a hand, Shaun?'

'If you've got a few moments, that'd be good. I'll take the head injury if you can check out Meredith's abdomen.' He was already focusing on the head, feeling for skull fractures.

Pulling on gloves, Nikki, with Georgie's help, slid Meredith's trousers down to expose the abdomen.

Behind her, a paramedic continued filling them in on details. 'The right thigh is tender to the touch, as is her right shoulder.'

'Did the car spin into the pole?' All the injuries seemed to be on one side, as though she'd been flung sideways.

'According to a bystander, yes.'

Glancing at Shaun, she found him looking at her. 'Makes sense?'

'It's the right side of her head that's taken the impact,' he agreed.

'Want me to alert the neurology department?'

'Yes, along with Radiology for X-rays and a CT scan. Orthopaedics too.' He returned to checking Meredith's head and neck.

'There's swelling at the top of the colon,' she told him as she ripped the gloves off. 'I'll be back shortly.' Getting specialists on the job was the priority.

Shaun sighed as Nikki strode away. She was the loveliest woman he'd encountered in a long time. Spending time with her during the weekend had been wonderful, and as for the sex—out of this world.

'Meredith, I'm going to check your shoulder. It's possibly dislocated, and this might hurt. Tell me if it's too much.' He didn't wait for an answer, got on with feeling the bones to see if they were in the right place. 'Not dislocated,' he said moments later. 'More likely a fracture.' Which meant another operation ahead.

He moved down the bed to Meredith's exposed abdomen and within moments agreed with Nikki. Now they needed to find the cause of the swelling. The upper bowel seemed fine. Then he touched the pancreas. Meredith cried out, making him feel bad. 'I'm sorry. Your pancreas appears to have ruptured. We'll know more after an X-ray of the abdominal area.'

Nikki was back, all professional and organised. Back straight, serious face on, organised to a T. Except he had his own special memories that were quite the opposite. Nikki all hot with her hair mussy as it spilled over the pillows. Her mouth soft and sensual as she tracked over his hot skin with her tongue. He reminded himself to concentrate as she said in a professional voice with a hint of a smile for him, 'An orderly's coming to take Meredith to Radiology as soon as the neurologist has been, and he's on his way down now. Someone from Orthopaedics will be along after Meredith's back from Radiology.'

'Thanks.' He'd wondered how she'd react towards him today. She seemed to like to keep her personal life to herself, and even being overly friendly might be going too far. At the moment, all was good. She wasn't making a big deal out of their time together, but neither was she ignoring him. A relief, really, because he liked her and didn't want to return to being only a colleague. He was settling down, and that meant making permanent friends. Friends like Nikki.

Looking around, he spied her talking to a little boy holding his arm hard against his chest. She was crouched down looking at the kid, touching his arm and asking questions, and the kid was answering her. She was good with the little ones. No doubt she'd make a great mother if that's what she wanted. He knew almost nothing about her. It was quite exciting in an odd way. Getting to know Nikki Marlow better would mean stepping outside his comfort zone. He could do it.

'Is this the patient with a head injury?' Charlie, a neurologist, asked from behind him.

Spinning around, Shaun nodded. 'Yes, Charlie, meet Meredith. She's been in a car accident where her right side seems to have taken the brunt of the impact.' He went on to describe the head injuries he'd found, all thoughts of Nikki on the back burner.

But she returned the moment he sent Meredith to Radiology with an orderly. 'Shaun, can you see to the elderly gentleman in cubicle six? He had a fall down some stairs during the night and couldn't move to get help. It was his grandson calling in on the way to school who found him and called 111.'

'A fall or a stroke?' Shaun wondered aloud as he headed for the cubicle.

'The paramedic thinks stroke. His speech is indistinct,' Nikki said from behind him. 'His name's Jason.'

'Hello, Jason. I'm Shaun, a doctor. I hear you got yourself into a bit of bother.' Shaun watched for the man's reactions.

'Y-yes.'

'Do you remember what happened?'

Jason moved his head awkwardly to one side. 'N-no.' His words were slurred. A stroke was a likely possibility.

'Okay, don't try to move at the moment. I'm going to touch your arm, then fingers and further down your body. If you feel me do that just say yes.' Shaun slipped up the sleeve of Jason's pyjama top and touched his bicep.

No reaction.

Same when he touched his wrist, then fingers. Whether that was because he hadn't felt anything or because he hadn't understood what Shaun had said didn't matter. He was going with the diagnosis of a stroke. 'We need oxygen. His breathing's shallow. I'll see if we've got a medical history for him.'

'The paramedic seemed to know him, which suggests he's been here before, though what for I've no idea,' Georgie answered. 'I'll fetch the oxygen and get that going.'

At the desk, Shaun looked up his patient and found he had been on blood thinners but had stopped taking them a month ago. 'Why?' There was no answer in the notes. Now he'd have to go back on them fast. There'd be clots in the man's blood system causing the stroke.

'Why what?' Nikki sat down at the computer next to him.

'The man stopped taking his dabigatran. It's in the notes but not the reason. His idea or the GP's?'

'I doubt it would've been his doctor's.'

'So do I.' Suddenly the air had a floral scent. Nikki's scent. Damn it. Now he'd smell her all day long, and with that would be the memories of what it had been like to get up close and personal to her satin-like skin. How was he going to get through the week if this was what she did to him within the first hour on duty?

She began filling in a prescription on the screen like she had no difficulty being near him.

He'd follow her example—because he didn't mind being near her. 'What's up with the little boy?'

Her smile illuminated the already well-lit area. 'Billy. He put his hand down a drain hole. When he tried to pull out, it was stuck, so he banged the drain with a stone to break it, and broke a bone in his wrist instead. It's not funny, but the kid is quite a character, saying he is going to be a plumber like his dad one day and was practising removing dirt from the drain.'

'He didn't seem too upset when he was talking to you.'

'No, the upset one would be Billy's mother.

She was shaking her head at him with worry in her eyes all the time he was telling me his story. I think she's got her hands full keeping an eye out for him.'

'Better than sitting glaring at a phone all day, I reckon.' Shaun stood up to return to Jason.

'Couldn't agree more.' Nikki went back to her screen, the smile still on her lips.

Thank goodness scrubs aren't tight-fitting was what he thought as he walked away. If that's all it took to make him start hardening, might be an idea to wear a bigger size from now on.

'Home sweet home,' Nikki muttered as she dropped her shoulder bag and the groceries she'd bought onto the bench and pulled the band off her ponytail. Shaking her hair about so it fell over her shoulders, she groaned. The day had gone on forever, and that wasn't only because of the number of patients that came into the ED.

Shaun had caught her attention from the moment he'd walked up behind her that morning and hadn't left her head since. It didn't help that they were often at the department hub at the same time, where she could not avoid noticing him, seeing that body filling out the scrubs and knowing exactly what they covered. As for the spicy aftershave smell, she was a goner. It'd been hard not to reach across and run her palm over the light bristle on his chin. She hadn't been a beard girl before, but the light one on Shaun's face stole the air out of her lungs. It was gorgeous and emphasised his good looks.

It was only Monday. Thankfully they'd got along fine. She'd been worried he might be overly friendly towards her, but there'd been no mention of the weekend, for which she was grateful. She didn't need other doctors or nurses knowing they'd spent time together. She'd also been concerned he might be a bit aloof if he didn't want to continue seeing her outside of work, but he hadn't. Seemed that they would carry on as they had last week until Saturday. All work and no play. Perfect.

Or it would be if she could ignore how happy she was whenever he was nearby. And warm in a special kind of way. And hot whenever she looked at his beard or smelled the aftershave.

Time for a wine. She'd earned it. The flow of patients hadn't slowed all day, mainly non-urgent cases but still needing total concentration. That was the only way she dealt with patients. It's what they deserved and what she loved giving them.

Laughter bubbled up as she thought about Billy. He was a right little man, cheeky and determined to be a plumber when he grew up, or way before then if today was anything to go by. If she had kids, she'd want them to be like that, confident and cute all in one. Like Shaun.

The wine sloshed over the side of the glass as

she poured. Shaun was not cute. He was too much of a man to be that. How about good-looking and sexy? Definitely. She'd been saying it to herself all day and needed to back off. There hadn't been any blips in their work relationship throughout the shift, but she couldn't start looking for more to what they had than was really there. It had been a good day hiking followed by a wonderful dinner and awesome sex. That did not mean there was more to come.

Did she want more? Taking a sip of her drink, she mulled it over. It would be wonderful to find a man who loved her for who she was and wouldn't leave her on a whim, or expect her to be obedient and do as she was told all the time like her father had. Whether Shaun was that man, she had no idea. All she knew was that she more than liked him. He intrigued her with his ability not to rave on about himself or ask questions of her that were too deep and personal to answer until she knew him better. More than that, he made her feel comfortable, plus intrigued about him. The fact she'd kissed him without thought on Saturday night and followed up with intense sex said a lot about where she was at, because she wasn't one for leaping into bed with just any man. She might've wanted to, but rarely had she followed through. Yet with Shaun, once she leaned in to kiss him, she hadn't considered pulling back at all and hadn't had a single regret since.

Except for worrying about working with him and if he'd make it awkward around other staff.

Okay, she wasn't totally comfortable with everything, but then, wasn't that normal when starting a new relationship? Was this already a relationship? She didn't think so but couldn't find another word to describe what they had going, or even if it would continue or had been a one-off, which was more likely. Shaun didn't seem in awe of her, she laughed sadly.

Time to stop this and do something practical. Like download the photos she'd taken on the hike and see if any of them were worth keeping.

As the lasagne she'd bought at the deli heated in the oven, she downloaded the photos onto her computer and studied them, looking for imperfections. There were plenty. The photos were good but not perfect, and she was a bit of a perfectionist when it came to her photography. It was why she'd won an award for one she took of a tui in some bushes by a beach last year.

She clicked through the photos, deleting some as she went. Her hand stopped as one appeared on the screen. Shaun stood on top of the hill where they'd had lunch, staring out over the valley, looking completely at ease with himself. Something, she realised, he didn't often appear to be. She'd known he enjoyed the walk but hadn't seen how truly relaxed he'd been. Why wasn't he like that more often? What had happened that kept him on edge? He had said his best friend had died, but not how or where. She was probably looking for something that wasn't there.

She couldn't drag her eyes away from the photo. No denying he was getting to her, and that she wasn't unhappy about it.

'Feel like a meal at the pub and then going to see a movie?' Nikki asked Shaun on Wednesday as they were making their way out to the car park at the end of shift. No matter how hard she'd tried, she hadn't been able to put last Saturday behind her and pretend she wanted nothing more to do with him. She named the movie she wanted to see.

Shaun didn't even hesitate. 'Beats grocery shopping any day. Add in how I'd thought about seeing that movie and you're on.'

Relief filled her. 'Great. Thought we'd go to the Jolly Roger pub. Shall I pick you up?'

'I'll meet you there. I've got to drop off some shoes for my nephews that my brother asked me to pick up.'

'So grocery shopping wasn't your plan?' She laughed, though it wasn't quite how she'd hoped to set up the evening. She'd still get to sit by him throughout the film and breathe in that aftershave that she enjoyed so much.

'Actually, I do need to get a few things, but they won't take long. See you at the pub around six?'

'Will do.' That gave her plenty of time for a long soak under the shower and finding the perfect shirt and jacket to wear with her new jeans. *Call me OTT, but I'm loving this dating stuff,* Nikki laughed to herself as she headed home with a skip in her step. Who'd have thought she'd be so relaxed about asking Shaun to go out for a meal with her? That feeling stayed with her throughout the evening.

'Those fish and chips were delicious.' Shaun pushed the plate aside and drained the last mouthful from his glass of beer.

'Not bad at all,' she agreed. 'Have you looked at any more houses lately?'

'A couple, but neither got me excited. It's harder to find what I like than I thought it would be.'

'You're not picky by any chance?' She grinned to show she didn't mean anything off by that.

'If wanting everything for nothing is picky, then I guess I am.' He chuckled. 'Seriously, I hadn't thought too much about what I might prefer. A house is a house, or so I thought.'

'When I decided to buy my own, I thought I wanted modern with little upkeep. Then one day I was heading over to Molly's when I saw an open home sign and on a whim stopped to look at the house. I was sold from the moment I walked inside.' The ambiance had grabbed her heartstrings. She probably paid too much, but nothing was stopping her buying the house.

'I have a feeling that's what I'm hoping for. A place I'll know immediately is my home.' Shaun checked his watch. 'We'd better get a wiggle on if we're not going to miss the beginning of the movie.'

She picked up the tab. 'My turn, and don't bother arguing.'

Shaun laughed. 'Me? Argue with you? I don't think so.'

'The movie was better than I'd expected,' Nikki said as they walked to their cars afterwards.

'I thought it was a bit drawn out, frankly.'

It was hard walking beside him and not grabbing his hand, but she managed. It was a casual date, and she was being careful not to set herself up for a fall. When they reached their vehicles, she said as casually as she could manage, 'See you tomorrow, bright and early.' No going back to her place for hot sexercise.

Shaun reached for her and placed a gentle kiss on her cheek. 'Early, maybe not so bright. Thanks for a lovely time.' He waited until she was in her car before he went to his. A true gentleman.

He didn't follow her home though. She should've been grateful but a part of her felt disappointed.

Then her phone lit up. Shaun. 'Hey.'

'How about a walk out Governors Bay way sometime over the weekend?'

'You're on.'

'Good. Sort details tomorrow. Bye.'

She did a wriggle in her seat. Woo-hoo. Another date with Shaun. Yes, they were dating. As friends or more, she didn't know, but she'd take what was on offer and enjoy every moment.

CHAPTER SEVEN

FRIDAY AT LAST and the end of shift. Shaun was looking forward to going hiking with Nikki again if she was still keen. Wednesday night at the pub and movies had been good, friendly without getting too intense. They hadn't returned to her bed for a repeat of the other night, which had to be for the best, for now, anyway. But he couldn't deny he could do with more time like that with her.

She was sitting in the hub, signing off for the day, looking as lovely as ever.

'Hey, Shaun, you got anything on tomorrow night?' Charlie, the neurologist, stepped in front of him.

'Nothing planned.' Though he had thought he'd ask Nikki to dinner if she was willing.

'How about coming to my place for dinner? I know it's short notice, but there's a small group of us who get together every month or so at one or other's house to relax and put work behind us for a while. You could get to know us a bit better without scrubs on.'

'Sounds good. What do I bring?'

'Whatever you like to drink. We take turns in either cooking or ordering in food. It's all very casual.'

'I'm in. Where do you live?' Who else would be there? Nikki?

'Give me your number and I'll text the address. Glad you've agreed to join us. Bring your partner if you've got one.' His eyebrow rose in a question mark.

'Nope. Just me.' At the moment. He'd ask Nikki if she wasn't already going, but that might be awkward when it was a group of colleagues getting together.

'No problem.'

It usually wasn't, but right now, he felt sad. He could ask Nikki if she was going and offer to pick her up. Or he could turn up alone. 'Here's my number,' he told Charlie.

'Thanks. See you tomorrow night, Nikki,' Charlie called out.

'Looking forward to it.'

His question answered, there was a lightness in Shaun's step as he made his way to the changing room. He was going to dinner at Charlie's, and Nikki would be there too. He was beginning to accept he wanted to spend time with her as friends, and maybe as more than that.

When Charlie's text with the address popped up on his phone, he saw Nikki lived only a couple of streets away from the neurosurgeon's. When he drove towards Charlie's on Saturday evening and saw Nikki walking along the street, he pulled over and opened the passenger window. 'Like a lift?'

'It would be rude to say no.'

Leaning across, he opened the door. 'That bag looks heavy.'

'Wine and books. Simone and I swap books all the time. She's Charlie's wife, in case you didn't know.'

'I didn't. I don't even know who else's going to be there.'

She turned to look at him and quickly filled him in. 'You've probably met them all apart from their other halves.'

Those drop-dead gorgeous eyes drew him in like an open fire on a cold winter's day. It was getting harder to stick to the friends idea. Even friends with benefits didn't quite gel. Time to let go and take a chance at happiness? It could be.

'Shaun? Hello?'

He shook his head and turned to face the front. He needed to get back on the road. 'Sorry. I was miles away. But I heard what you said,' he added quickly.

'That I don't like dogs?'

'You didn't say that?' Had she? 'No, you said you like them when I mentioned I might get one once I've bought a house.'

Her laugh teased him. 'Just jibbing you because you looked so far away for a moment.'

He'd been right here with her. 'Let's go.' He wasn't getting any deeper into this quagmire than he already was. She'd think he was crazy and want to get out of the car to start walking again.

'First street on the left.'

'I've got it. Used to spend quite a bit of time around here when I was at high school as some of my mates lived in this area.' Liam for one. He could picture the dude giving him the thumbs-up for spending more time with Nikki.

'What's it like returning home after years away? Are your friends still around, or have they moved away?'

So much for thinking she wouldn't ask personal questions, though to be fair, it wasn't a deep one. 'A couple are here. Others have gone for their work or to their partners' towns. Most importantly, my family's here. I missed them more than anyone when I was away.' Now who was getting a little deeper into his background? 'It doesn't seem to matter where I am or what I'm doing. They're always a part of my life, even if it's to tell me I'm making a mistake about something I've done.'

'That's families, I guess.' There was a longing in her voice.

'Not like yours?'

'My brother, definitely. Mum, not so much.'

He wanted to ask about her father, but she was closing down, and that was the last thing he needed. No, actually, they were friends. He could ask. 'What about your father?'

'He died a few years ago. He wasn't the best dad out there.'

There was so much he wanted to know, but the pain in her voice put the dampener on that. 'Which station does your brother work out of?'

'Christchurch Central.'

'That must keep him busy.'

'It does, but not so much that he's not there for his family. They come first, no matter what.'

Turning into Charlie's street, he looked along the road. 'We're headed where all those cars are parked?'

'You're on to it.' Nikki rolled her shoulders. 'Thanks for this.'

'It's cold out there. I'll take you home afterwards.'

'I could get to like you.' She laughed.

'You don't already?'

'Yeah, okay, like you even more.'

'That's better.' It was silly talk, but she was lightening up again, and that made him happy.

'What about going for that walk you mentioned tomorrow morning?' she asked as he parked on the side of the road.

The one he hadn't done anything about because caution had won—for a while at least. 'I guess we could.'

But was it a good idea if he wanted to stay safe from temptation? *Come on. Get over your hang-ups.* Time with Nikki was always wonderful.

'Fine. Obviously you're not keen anymore.' She opened her door.

He reached for her arm, held her lightly. 'Sorry, I'd like to go for one.' The kids, sports. Damn. 'I'm going to watch my nephews play soccer at ten. Want to join me, and then we could do a shorter walk after?'

'What?' Her eyes widened in surprise.

He felt the same. He'd just asked her to meet his family. That was left field, if ever anything was, and totally out of sync with being cautious. 'If you can put up with two toe-rags giving you cheek, that is.'

'That's a challenge I can't refuse.'

'So I figured.' He hadn't thought that at all, but hey, she was going with him, so all was good. Better than he'd planned on.

Nikki pinched herself. Did Shaun really suggest she join him with his nephews in the morning? He was beginning to open up to her. He wasn't withdrawing as she'd been thinking. Woo-hoo. Bring it on. These past weeks, she'd done little but think about Shaun and how he made her feel special without even trying. Despite all the warnings going off in her head about how Brett had also once made her feel special, she knew the time had come to take some risks. She did not want to look back and regret a missed opportunity at happiness. If she was getting carried away with the idea, then so be it. Right now it was hard to deny how comfortable she was with Shaun. Even knowing he was right to leave her place last Saturday night, she couldn't stop feeling this going well.

He walked into Charlie's house beside her. 'I'm looking forward to this.'

'Good, because everyone's great company.' As she glanced at Shaun, her heart moved. Yes, he was special. Hopefully she could come to be special for him too.

Charlie spotted them instantly. 'Hi, you two. Come through and meet everyone, Shaun. I think you've met everyone except Sheree. She's a radiologist. Nikki, Simone's in the wine cellar looking for some Pinot Gris that's supposedly better than the one I brought up.'

'I'll go help her.' When she found what she was looking for, Simone wouldn't bring only one or two bottles up from the chiller. Never mind that everyone usually brought a bottle with them. She liked being generous. 'You got this, Shaun?'

'You bet.' He gave her the cheeky smile that did nothing to calm her.

Instead it fired up the hormones he'd wreaked

havoc with two weeks ago. Grand. They'd been here barely two minutes and already she was in a mess over him. She placed her bag on the hall table before disappearing down the stairs to the cellar. Here she breathed, hoping to calm her hormones. 'Hey, Simone, I hear you're looking for a certain wine.'

The walk-in chiller was open, and Simone was inside, reading labels on numerous bottles. 'Not having much luck, I'm afraid. Must've finished it when the family were here for my birthday last month.'

'Doesn't matter. I've brought Pinot Gris and Chardonnay.' Not all for her.

'Thanks. I so wanted you all to try that particular one. Never mind, let's get back upstairs and join in the fun. Charlie says he invited Shaun Elliott from ED along.'

She nodded. 'He started with us three weeks ago.'

'How's he doing?'

'He's great. Just who we needed.' Surely her cheeks weren't warming in the cool air of the chiller? How embarrassing.

'You like him.'

More than embarrassing. 'Of course.'

'I don't mean as a colleague. It does happen, you know. Doctors fall for other doctors or nurses all the time. Take Charlie and me, for example. We met at Wellington Hospital nine years ago and haven't been apart since.' Simone was an obstetrician.

'Steady up. You know I'm ultra-cautious when it comes to men and relationships.'

Simone gave her a quick hug. 'Maybe it's time to have some fun and fall in love along the way.'

'You're an old nag.'

'But a good one. Come on, let's grab a glass of wine, and I can suss out this guy who makes you blush far too easily.'

She had no answer to that. 'Bring on the wine.' Nothing else.

It wasn't easy to avoid Shaun when the moment she stepped into the lounge he smiled directly at her, once more tightening her insides. Those blue eyes were always drawing her in and making her feel a part of him. He really was a problem—a good problem, she admitted. Seeing Shaun so relaxed, she pictured a little boy looking just like him. 'Where're the wine glasses?' she demanded of Simone.

'Got it that bad, huh?'

'Oh, shut up.' She really was letting Shaun get to her in far too many ways.

Simone laughed out loud, which had everyone looking their way. 'Which would you like? Pinot Gris or Chardonnay?'

Both. Pour me a bucketful. 'Chardonnay, thanks.'

'I'll get those.' Shaun was right there. 'I'm

Shaun, by the way.' He held his hand out to Simone. 'Charlie's wife?'

'That's me. I'm glad you've joined us. I'm sure you'll have a lovely night.' At least she didn't look at Nikki when she said it.

Nikki sighed. There was no getting away from Simone, so she'd concentrate on talking about boring subjects, and hopefully she'd back off.

Shaun handed Nikki her Chardonnay and a Pinot Gris to Simone, then raised his glass. 'Cheers. Here's to a great evening. It's already turning out to be fun. Everyone's so relaxed and easy to talk to.'

'What did you expect?'

'From past experience, sometimes there can be a bit of one-upmanship at these dos.'

She'd never struck that. 'Might be you're out of practice.'

'True. It helps me feel like I'm starting to fit in, something I haven't bothered with too much lately. When I was only ever in any place for a few months, I never put a lot of effort into getting to know my colleagues out of work.'

'Sounds lonely.' He could be congenial with everyone and yet cautious about mixing with people as well. Other than her. He seemed keen to spend time with her. She didn't think the walking was all about keeping fit. He didn't need her for that, but she understood the loneliness.

'I won't lie. It was at times. Part of returning home means finding friends.'

What about me? She swallowed a big mouthful of wine and started coughing.

Shaun instantly patted her back hard enough to ease the coughing. 'Easy, girl.'

She laughed. 'Girl? Not for a while now.'

He laughed too. 'You think?'

'Hey, you two. Get over here and tell us what's so funny,' Paul called across the room.

'I was pointing out to Nikki she shouldn't be wearing high heels when she's racing down stairs. It's not a good look to land head first at the bottom.'

'Careful, man. She'll have you on the floor with a judo hold in a flash if you're not careful.'

Shaun spun around to stare at her. 'You do judo?'

She burst out laughing. As if she was going to spend time getting thrown to the floor or returning the favour with someone else. 'Welcome to the group, Shaun.'

He grinned. 'Guess I got that one wrong. Let me know if you ever want to find out what it's like to be dropped to the mat in a bundle.'

She gaped at him. 'What belt have you got?'

'A faded green one.' His grin was still in place, wreaking havoc with her head and heart. 'I gave up when I left school to go to university. Far more interesting things to discover there.'

'Beer and girls,' Charlie agreed.

'You're on to it.' Shaun wandered closer to the others, at the same time making sure she came with him. 'Nikki dragged me out on one of the tracks on Mount Richardson a couple of weekends ago. It was good to do something else I haven't done in ages.'

So much for not letting people know they'd seen each other outside work. No one looked surprised, or even shocked. More like they were pleased that she and Shaun had done something together. That rocked her. While some of them were brutally honest about their thoughts on her not dating more often, she wouldn't have expected them to think she should go out with the new doctor in the department. 'His boots were very dusty.'

'We're thinking about heading up to Hanmer Springs for a weekend next month,' Simone said. 'Those of us who aren't on call, that is. There're walks around there if you're interested, Shaun.'

'I could be, depending on the roster and when you decide to go.'

'We'll keep you posted.'

He'd been accepted into the group. Nikki wasn't sure if that was good for her or not. Fine while they were getting on, not so much if they fell out. There again, she was trying to move forward with this, and thinking about things going wrong wasn't the way to do it. 'Better polish those boots,' she said with a laugh.

'Done that already.'

'Dinner's ready in five if anyone needs to top up their glass beforehand,' Simone said.

Nikki, along with Sheree and Mallory, Paul's wife, headed for the kitchen to give her a hand putting food on serving dishes and taking them to the long table in the dining room. This was a normal evening with friends, and yet she felt a new buzz in her veins. Shaun. He had a way about him that lifted her concerns regarding her future that she couldn't ignore. He was special.

'Stop smiling so much.' Simone grinned. 'You'll have everyone thinking he's already had his way with you.'

Heat scorched her cheeks.

'Oh, oh. I see. Well done, girlfriend.'

'Simone, shut up.'

She laughed. 'Okay.' She returned to plating up the broccoli and pecan salad.

Mallory and Sheree were grinning too. No secrets with this lot.

Then Nikki found herself laughing. She'd had some lovely times with Shaun and felt lighter in spirit for them. 'What the heck?'

'What's mentioned at dinner stays at dinner,' Sheree said.

'You know he's worked in Christchurch ED before?' Mallory asked.

'I heard that. Why did he leave?' Was he restless back then too?

'Do you remember when a pilot of a small plane died while in the air and his passenger landed the plane with no flying experience? It was about four years ago.'

'Vaguely. I was in Auckland back then.' Was Mallory talking about Shaun?

'Well, Shaun was the man who brought the plane down. Amazing feat considering. His friend had had a fatal heart attack.'

Nikki's heart slumped. The mate who'd died. 'Oh.' She was lost for words.

Mallory nudged her. 'You haven't heard it from me, okay? I don't normally gossip, but I wanted to give you the facts, brief as they are.'

'Thanks, Mallory. It explains a few things.'

'Stop frowning. You'll get wrinkles on your forehead.'

'Come on, let's eat,' Simone said and carried the last platters into the dining room.

'Nikki, how's your glass?' Shaun asked the moment she entered the dining room.

'Almost empty.' Normally she wouldn't have more than one drink, but right now it seemed like a good idea to have another. She finished the wine and handed Shaun the glass. 'Thanks.'

Of course Simone made sure she and Shaun were sitting together at the table. If asked, they'd probably say that was because the two of them were on their own, so it was the natural thing to do, but Nikki knew there was some stirring going on. At least everyone was okay about her and Shaun being together and not looking for trouble. Another thing to be grateful for.

'Would you like some gurnard?' Shaun held a platter with baked fish towards her.

'You bet. What about you? Like seafood?'

'Can't get enough of it.'

'You into fishing by any chance?' Paul asked. 'None of these morons like getting smelly handling the bait.'

'Anytime you need someone to go out with you, give me a call.'

'You're on.'

He look so relaxed and happy, Nikki couldn't help smiling. It wasn't as though he was a surly man, more that he didn't often open up around people. She was beginning to understand why. He'd been through hell. That made her feel closer to him and hope there'd be more occasions for him to enjoy, some with her. She wanted Shaun to stay in Christchurch permanently. She really and truly did. He was showing her she could let go of her fears and enjoy life more than she had since breaking up with her ex. Hopefully she might be able to return the favour.

Hours later, Shaun pulled into Nikki's driveway and cut the motor. Should he stay a while? Or would it be wiser to head home before they got too involved? Except he wanted to spend more time with Nikki. Lots more, scary as that might be. 'That was a great night.'

'Certainly was,' Nikki responded with a smile. 'They're a good bunch. It's fun seeing a side to them that's got nothing to do with sick or injured people.'

'Reminds you that you're more than a doctor?' He got that in spades. Being a medic was a serious job, though there were light moments when patients cracked jokes or could finally get out of bed and walk by themselves once more. But to be able to fully relax and not think about the consequences of being himself with other people who understood was great. 'How long have you been a part of the group?'

'From when I came to Christchurch. After I split up with my husband.'

So Nikki had been married before. 'You're divorced?'

'Yes.' The word ground out through her teeth before she turned to look at him. 'I had a miscarriage. Brett left to live with his girlfriend who was also pregnant and needed his support, since I was no longer having a baby. Unbeknown to me, they'd been having an affair for many months. He's a GP with a practice in Auckland, and she was a nurse working for him. All those nights he told me he was seeing patients, he was actually having sex with her.' That beautiful smile was gone.

He reached over and wrapped her in his arms. 'How did you cope? I mean, how could he leave you when you'd be grieving for your baby? I don't get it.'

'Seems I didn't know him as well as I thought.'

'Nikki, my heart's breaking for you. How did you get out of bed every morning?'

'Slowly.'

'I bet.' But she had got up. No surprise there. 'Did you seek help? Talk to anyone?'

Lifting her head, she stared at him for a long moment. 'Yes.'

'That man had better not come visiting any time or there'll be trouble.'

'No, there won't. You'd be there for anyone you believed needed you, but you'd never do what you're implying.'

The air whooshed out of his lungs. Nikki had just said something amazing to him, about him. He wouldn't have expected that in a million years. 'Thanks,' he croaked.

'Come on. Let's go inside.' That wasn't an invitation, more of an insistence with a small smile thrown in.

One he was happy to comply with. 'Thought you'd never ask.' She wanted done with this conversation, and he'd comply. Having her drag up any more painful memories wouldn't be fun.

'Coffee, wine or me?' she asked as she closed the door behind them.

He looked at her, saw the amazing, strong woman she was along with the doubt in her eyes. He still had no idea where he was going with this and didn't want to get in so deep he couldn't get out, but neither did he want to ignore her doubt. She needed him at the moment. He enfolded her in his arms. 'You.'

They stood there embracing each other for a long, quiet moment before he swept her up and strode to her bedroom to place her on the bed, then knelt down to kiss her smile. Followed by her chin, neck and down the wonderful cleavage he knew was behind the cream blouse. All the time her fingers were working hot, sexy magic on his skin, arousing him way too fast. 'Stop,' he said, panting.

'Soon,' she whispered.

'Soon will be too late.'

'You think?'

'I know.'

Then there was no thinking going on. Their bodies melded into each other as their mouths met. Clothes flew through the air as they hurriedly undressed. And then Nikki was as naked as it was possible to be.

He drank in the beautiful sight. She really was something else. He could fall in love if he wasn't careful. But he was always careful, so he was safe, despite how his heart was beating hard and erratically.

'Shaun?' Doubt was creeping into her face.

'Coming.' Lying on the bed, he wrapped her in his arms and legs. 'I meant—'

'You're coming.' The doubt was replaced by a sexy-as-hell twinkle in her eyes. 'Me too.'

They didn't say anything else. Their bodies took over their minds and led them on an amazing ride.

Sometime later, Shaun woke to find Nikki curled up against him, her arm tight around his waist. The sense of belonging was strong. They got along so well he could accept his plans for coming home might all work out.

Nikki had been hurt by that low-life of a husband. How could he have an affair, especially when she'd been carrying his child? He'd got the other woman pregnant too. Nikki deserved so much better. Hearing why her marriage ended made Shaun seethe. She must feel so vulnerable now. Was that why she didn't talk about her past and her feelings? Like him not talking about his. They were both protecting their hearts. Was that why she agreed with him when he'd said he was going home the other night? She didn't want to be hurt again.

Gazing at her sleeping against him, he felt a longing he hadn't known since Amy begin to spread throughout him and raise his protective instincts for Nikki. Which said he might be getting too close, too soon. Although he thought the world of her and did want a proper relationship further down the track, he did not want to rush things. It was time to go home, put space between them. Staying through till morning suggested he'd like more than a brief get-together in bed, and he didn't want to give Nikki the wrong idea about where he stood at the moment. That could hurt her, and that wasn't happening as far as he was concerned.

Slowly and quietly he slipped out of bed, doing his damnedest not to wake her. Once dressed he made for the door, then turned back. No way could he walk out of the room without placing a tender kiss on her soft lips. Leaning over, he did just that, holding his breath, still not wanting to wake her.

'Shaun?' she croaked, one eye dragging open.

'Shh, go back to sleep. See you later,' he whispered. 'I promise,' he added so she knew he wasn't running away from what they were sharing.

Her eye closed, and she snuggled into her pillow. Gorgeous. As tempting as it was to climb back in with her, he headed away. Time to be play sensible. For a while anyway.

'Shh, go back to sleep,' Shaun had whispered in her ear during the night.

Now he wasn't here.

Nikki stretched full-length in her bed. She'd slept in. The sun was streaming in around the edges of the curtains where she hadn't closed them completely. After walking around the park yesterday morning plus an entertaining evening with her friends and then making out with Shaun, she'd been tired. Throw in the busy week, and it was no wonder she hadn't woken at her usual time.

'Why did you go home, Shaun?' They could've had breakfast together before watching the boys play soccer. Then again, they weren't partners or in a relationship of any kind, other than a few outings together and amazing sex. But she liked him more than a lot and wanted to spend more time with him.

So it was just as well he'd gone home. He mightn't be keen while she was getting too keen. She'd reached a point where she felt ready to take a chance on settling down with a man if she loved him, yet she still worried about being hurt. Moving on from Brett had been hard. She'd loved him so much. After her childhood never living in one place for long, a man who said he loved her and wanted to live with her forever in one place was a keeper. Putting him behind her and getting back out dating when she understood that people made promises they had no intention of keeping had been a struggle.

Yet along came Shaun, and the barriers around her heart began dropping away fast. *Too fast, Nikki.* That was the problem. Because she wanted to let him in, at least enough to get to know him for real, and be certain he was the right man for her before making a big mistake.

Tossing the duvet aside, she clambered out of bed and grinned at the new aches. Her body had had quite a workout, showing how out of practice she was. Yes, this was definitely going well, and she could relax about him disappearing after they had sex. He was probably protecting himself as much as she was herself.

A long, hot shower put her on top of the world again. Add a strong coffee and marmalade-covered toast and she was ready for just about anything. Looking outside, she sighed. 'Darn, the lawns need cutting.' Not her favourite pastime for sure.

The phone rang. 'Saved.'

Shaun. 'Nikki, did you sleep in?'

'I did. How about you?' It would've been bliss snuggled up to that hot body as she came awake.

'No, I've been for a run. The boys' soccer's been cancelled. They're going to a birthday party instead. But I was wondering if you'd do something else with me. Not the walk.'

'I was looking forward to meeting your family.'

'I need to look at an open home and wondered if you'd come with me. I saw the house on Thursday and liked it a lot, but I want another opinion if you're up for it.'

She wasn't going to meet his family? That stung, even when there was a good reason not to. She'd felt like he'd been opening a door for her, and now it had been slammed shut again. But then, he wanted her to look at a house he was interested in. Could he be taking their friend-ship another step? He hadn't mentioned anything about looking at houses last night. She could give him some leeway and see where it led. 'Beats mowing the lawns any time.'

His laughter warmed her through and through. 'I'm not picking you up for a few hours. You've got plenty of time.'

'Spoil-sport.' He was right, though, and now she was going to see him later, it didn't seem so much of a hassle to get the mower out and do the job. 'See you soon.'

She almost skipped around the lawn. It had never been so quick to mow the lawns. After shoving the mower back into the corner of the garage, she locked the door and went inside for another shower. Not that she really needed one but she liked to be ready in case they got all hot and close again.

'Where's this house?' Nikki asked when Shaun arrived to pick her up.

'Merivale. Perfect for work and not far from family.' His fingers were tapping the steering wheel. 'The owners are moving up to Napier for family reasons and are looking for a quick sale.' There was a lightness in his voice that suggested he was keener than he'd let on.

'Is it in good nick? Or is there work to be done?'

'It's perfect. Just walk in and get on with life.'

Interesting. So he *was* staying, or at least working at making it happen. That looked good for the future. In lots of ways, not only because she was starting to let him in but because he might finally find what he was looking for. It was hard to accept when she was afraid of being left behind. Or being dragged from town to city to town. She'd put her own roots down here, but if she fell in love, then those roots might amount to nothing, and that frightened her.

He hadn't finished. 'I'd change the décor, though. It's all white, and I find that quite sterile. But I'm getting ahead of myself. This second viewing might reveal things I won't like about the property.'

'Then there's my opinion to consider,' she said with a laugh.

'There is that.'

'Seriously, you're not to listen to me if you think it's the house for you.'

'I won't.'

So why had he asked her to come along and

give her opinion? Was it a kind of date? 'You know I'll be honest about what I think?'

'Exactly why I'm taking you with me.' He chuckled. 'I thought I'd like someone to look at it and know what I might be letting myself in for. Buying a house is part of my plan for returning home.'

'You are determined to stay.'

'Why wouldn't I be?' he asked tightly. 'It's time to settle down in one place, and besides, my family is here.'

Ouch. Seemed that she'd touched a subject he didn't want to talk about. Was this to do with losing his friend years back? If so, she did feel bad for upsetting him. 'I imagine it won't be easy to stop moving around on a regular basis. Before you ask, I did hear that you'd been working in quite a few different locations lately.'

'I take it that Paul told you.'

'When I asked where you'd been working, all he said was that you'd been on the move a bit since leaving Christchurch General a few years ago. Nothing else. It was a normal question to ask about a new doctor coming on board.' Any minute now, he'd turn around and take her back home. 'I wasn't trying to pry.' After that reaction, she wasn't mentioning the loss of his friend. 'Nor was Paul speaking out of turn. He'd never blab about someone.'

Turning to face her, he said, 'I know. Sorry I overreacted.'

It wasn't like the Shaun she was coming to know, though she guessed she didn't really know him well at all. She was intrigued to find out what type of house piqued his interest. 'I've already forgotten what you said.'

Silence fell between them. It was the first time she'd felt uncomfortable with him, and she didn't like it. It wasn't as though she'd asked something deep and meaningful, surely? Whatever the reason, he didn't have to go quiet on her. She wasn't looking for trouble. Trouble was one thing she tried hard to avoid. Along with falling in love. Often the two went hand in hand.

When Shaun pulled into the driveway of a very modern-looking house with a large for-sale sign at the front, Nikki gasped. 'It's stunning.' Obviously someone had spent a small fortune to have an architect draw up the plans; the house hadn't been one of a building company's array of fast builds. 'The black framework highlights all those windows.'

'Which look directly onto the street,' Shaun commented. 'Though the current owners have planted a lot of shrubs that are beginning to break the view so that people walking past won't be able to peek in as much.'

'I can't wait to see inside.'

'Then let's do it. I'm liking your positive vibes so far.' Shaun was smiling again.

The tension gripping her faded away. 'You couldn't have more different taste in houses than me.' Nothing like her little old cottage, but she'd never expected to fall in love with it either.

A well-dressed woman, presumably the real estate agent, stepped out onto the terrace. 'Hello, Shaun. The owners have gone for a coffee while you have a look around. I'll stay here, out of your way.'

'Thanks. This is my friend, Nikki Marlow.'

Nikki shook the woman's hand. 'I'm looking forward to this.'

'Take your time. I'm not in a hurry to be any-where else.' The agent left them to wander inside on their own.

Looking around as she followed Shaun, Nikki shook her head. 'It's wonderful. Though I do agree there's too much white.'

'Easily fixed.'

'Do you really think grey?' She felt more co-lour was needed, but then, she could be way out of tune with the latest fashion in house decora-tions.

'I haven't come up with an answer to that yet. That's for when—if—I buy the place.'

'Fair enough.' A warm green came to mind. She'd keep that to herself. This wasn't going to be her home, even if she and Shaun were getting along just fine. They weren't likely to become more than friends with benefits for a long while, if at all. Too hard to let go the restraints she'd put on herself when he didn't have a good reputation for settling down. He might be looking to buy a house, but that didn't mean he was staying put from now on. He could always rent it out.

'What do you think?' Shaun asked after they'd had a thorough look around inside and out.

'I really like it. There's a certain wow factor about the whole property that kind of sucks me in a bit.'

'I know what you mean. Which is why I'm going to put in an offer.'

Nikki spun around to high-five him. 'Go you.' It was a step towards staying in Christchurch permanently, and she wouldn't be discouraging that even if she did have doubts about him staying long-term. It was her past and her father's continual moving from place to place that made her reluctant to believe Shaun could be different, not Shaun himself. She wanted to believe in him, wanted to think he was different and ready to change his lifestyle.

His smile was huge. 'Thanks for your support. It means a lot.'

She was grateful he hadn't been able to read her thoughts. 'Why don't you go discuss things with the agent, and I'll find my own way home.' She wasn't going to hang around while he got down and serious about his offer with the agent and how he was going to pay for it. That was his business and nothing to do with her.

'I can drop you home first.'

'No need. I'll walk over to the mall to get some film for my camera and then grab a taxi.'

'That seems unfair considering I asked you to come along to tell me what you thought about the property.'

'Go talk to the agent. I'm a big girl and can look after myself.' Leaning in, she placed a light kiss on his raspy chin. 'Good luck. Keep me posted.' She headed away before he could say anything else. But as she walked out of the drive, she peeked over her shoulder and found he was watching her, his finger touching his cheek where she'd kissed him. Warmth stole through her. He was special. And despite everything Brett had done, wakening her to all sorts of possibilities.

CHAPTER EIGHT

'HAVE YOU HEARD anything about how the legalities are going on your contract to buy the house?' Nikki asked as she looked hungrily at the eggs Benedict the server had just put before her. They looked yummy. When Shaun suggested breakfast over the road from the hospital at Suzie's when they came off night shift, she'd all but grabbed his hand and run across, she was that hungry.

He handed her the pepper grinder. 'Not a lot. The lawyer's still waiting for the council's building report. Apparently it usually takes at least a week so can't be far off.'

'Have you started looking at furniture yet?' He'd said he didn't have any, so it was going to be a big buy-up at some point.

'I had a wander around one of the big furniture stores. There was so much selection it was mind-blowing. I didn't know where to start, so I walked out.' He looked embarrassed.

'Not as easy as dealing with a drunk teen with

a broken leg then?' That had been one of his patients last night.

He grimaced. 'Put it like that and I sound hopeless.'

'Not at all. If you need a hand, give me a call. I have a thing about good furniture.'

'I might just do that.'

Really? If she had any doubts, that'd show how well they were getting on. She took a mouthful of eggs and sighed contentedly. Perfect. 'Just what the doctor ordered.'

'Not bad, are they?'

'What are you are up to today? Other than grabbing some sleep?'

'Having a round of golf with Dad. He's determined to make me improve my score, which is pretty bad, I admit. But I haven't had much practice at it.'

'Do you enjoy playing?' Somehow she wouldn't have thought golf was his thing.

'So-so. But it means I spend time with Dad, so I'm up for it, along with the ribbing I get about my lack of style.'

From the little he'd said, family meant a lot to Shaun. As Ross did to her. Not so much her parents, but that was history, and she wasn't wasting time wishing she could change it. 'Make the most of it,' she said.

Shaun nodded. 'I am.'

'Good.' A wave of sadness caught her. She and

Ross had missed out on so much growing up. She grabbed her coffee and took a gulp. But Ross had got his act together and was a wonderful father. She could do the same if she ever was lucky enough to have children. Glancing at Shaun, she felt flustered. She was stepping outside her barriers, and it was so darned scary. There was a lot to lose—or a lot to gain. Plastering a smile on her face before he noticed she was at odds with herself, she said, 'I can't imagine swinging a club at a ball and getting it to land in a tiny hole.'

'You want to try?'

'No, thanks.' Would he offer to show her how it's done? She'd turn him down on that one.

'Fair enough.' Shaun pushed his empty plate aside. 'So, what's on your agenda today?'

'Not a lot.' She hadn't made any plans. 'Might take the camera to Hagley Park and get some shots of the Avon River flowing through the greenery.' Actually, that's exactly what she'd do. Then she'd stop worrying about everything else.

'Another calendar in the making?' He'd been impressed with the one of birds she'd given him after their first walk.

'Who knows? It could be.' Anything was possible. *Get that, Nikki? Anything's possible.* She smiled. *Here's hoping.*

The following Friday, Shaun stared at the papers his lawyer handed him.

'Here you go,' she said. 'Sign these and the house is yours.'

Really? As in, he really had bought a house? The papers shook in his hand. Had he seriously ticked off another box on his list? There weren't many to go. Only one major one. The one he was not ready for, but getting closer.

'Shaun? You okay?'

He nodded. 'Yes.' Damn it, he truly was. This was the most exciting thing he'd done in forever, and his body was humming. With a firm hand, he signed on the line. 'I've bought a house. My own home. If I seem a little stunned, it's because I'm still absorbing what's happened.'

'I've seen it all before. There's something special about buying your first house.'

It wasn't his first. He and Amy had bought one on the other side of Christchurch when they got married. A little doer-upper that they'd enjoyed because it was *their* home. Once they decided to go their separate ways, neither of them wanted it—too many memories—so sold it. That had been a sad day for both of them. Now he had a new property to make his home. Life was looking up big-time. 'As long as I'm not getting ahead of myself,' he muttered.

If only Nikki was here to share this moment with him. He'd like that even if he was expecting too much when they weren't that close. Getting there, but they had a way to go—if he allowed it to happen. Right now, despite how happy he was, he wasn't sure what he felt about Nikki other than he seemed to be falling for her a little more as each week passed.

He needed to share his news with someone, and the first name to pop into his head was Nikki's. What about his parents? Or brother, or sister? No, the urge to call Nikki was stronger. So much for keeping her at arm's length.

Once outside the lawyer's office, he pulled his phone from his pocket and pressed her number.

'Hey, Shaun, what's up?'

Her voice thrilled him. Soft and caring all in one. He paused, wanting to drag out the moment, enjoying every second. This was so exciting.

Nikki waited.

The words burst out. 'The house is mine.'

'Woo-hoo. That's wonderful news.'

'Honestly, Nikki, I am thrilled. It's a wonderful property, and I can't wait to take over.'

'When's that likely to happen?'

'Two weeks from today. The current owners have already started packing as they're desperate to get to Napier.' Two weeks and he'd be moving into his own home. 'I've got a lot of shopping to do before then.' When he and Amy bought their place, they'd had to be cautious about what they spent. He'd put a lot of money away since then, always on the move and not filling any apartment with furniture he'd have to move whenever he headed to the next job. He'd also earned good wages with the shortage of doctors currently a problem for most health boards in the country. This was so much fun.

'Right. Unless you already have plans, I'm taking you out to dinner tonight to celebrate your news.'

His heart squeezed. Awesome. 'I'd like that more than anything else.' Now wasn't the time to keep Nikki at a distance. He couldn't. He was so happy to have bought a home and added a massive tick to his list that he could share the fun with someone special. Yes, Nikki was special, and becoming more so all the time. Another squeeze under his ribs. Right now he was a very happy man. Such a new feeling, and he was going to make the most of it. 'What time?'

'I'll pick you up just before seven.'

'I can pick *you* up.'

'No. It's your celebration, and you might want an extra drink or two. See you later.' Click. She was gone.

Five minutes later, he got a text from her. What's your address?

Laughing, he sent the details, ignoring the temptation to say now he had to pick *her* up. No point in stirring up trouble. Not that he believed she'd get cross, but still. Best to play fair and keep onside. Who knew how they might fill in the rest of the evening after dinner. Though he had a darned good idea of how he'd like to. No denying Nikki was beautiful and sexy and downright cool to be with. What was it about her that had him thinking like that? No woman since Amy had interested him half as much. He hadn't wanted them to, yet Nikki just wandered into his head and took over. Even his heart sometimes got a bit soft around her. Scary. Exciting. He truly was settling down and moving forward.

The evening was better than good. It was perfect. 'Dinner was amazing,' he told Nikki as they strolled hand in hand along the Avon River afterwards, wrapped in warm jackets. It was chilly, but the night sky was clear and full of twinkling stars. 'I've always enjoyed Spanish cuisine, but that was way beyond anything I've had before.'

'Glad you liked it. I wasn't sure if you would and did think of calling to ask, then decided to hell with it. If you didn't like Spanish food, then tough.' She laughed.

He paused and pulled her to a stop before drawing that delightful body in against his. 'Thanks for a great ending to a great day.'

'We had to celebrate. It's not every day you do something as important and exciting as buying a house.' She sounded almost as excited for him as he was.

'It's a big step.' He grinned. 'One I'm pleased I've made.' He was getting on with his plans. It *was* good, he told himself. So now he'd make the most of any time spent with Nikki and possibly grow the relationship further. Enjoying each other's company wasn't something to be tossed aside like a banana skin.

Leaning back in his arms, she locked her eyes with his. 'You mean that, don't you?'

It was a serious question he hadn't expected. 'Yes, Nikki, I do. I am determined to settle down here.'

After staring at him for a long moment, she placed her mouth on his. 'Good.' Then she kissed him hard.

He responded just as hard. She was hot and tasty, and other parts of him were hardening too. Jerking his head back, he growled, 'Nikki, can we go back to your place? Now?'

Her eyes widened as she gave him a wicked grin. 'What a good idea.'

It was hard to focus on driving with Shaun sitting next to her, Nikki thought. His hand on her thigh sent warm tremors throughout her, waking her body up and filling her with eager anticipation. Making love with Shaun had become her favourite pastime, and she couldn't get enough. There was a large hotel up ahead. It'd be too easy to pull in and grab a room for the night. Even though they were only ten minutes from her house, it would be fun going to a hotel with Shaun for a couple of hours.

'Pull in there.' Shaun nodded towards the hotel.

On the same page as her? A trickle of excitement raced down her spine. He was awesome. Indicating a right turn, Nikki crossed the road and pulled up outside the entrance, where the doorman opened Shaun's door.

'Good evening, sir. Do you have a booking with us? Or would you like to make one?'

'I'm going to see if a room is available.' Shaun hadn't leapt out of the car, was instead trying to adjust his trousers without being obvious.

Nikki giggled. 'I'll go in.'

'No, I'll take care of this.'

'There're rooms available.' The doorman spoke very politely, not a hint of a laugh anywhere on his face. He was probably used to couples turning up and being in a hurry for a bed. As they didn't have bags, it would be obvious what this was about, and for once she couldn't care less what the man thought. 'I'll park your car in the basement, madam.'

'Thank you.' Nikki got out and went around to Shaun. 'Ready?' She grinned.

'As I'll ever be.' He grinned back, standing up.

She winked. His situation wasn't quite so obvious as it had been. Could be that talking to the doorman had been a little like ice on his need.

Something for her to rectify the moment they were behind closed doors. Melt the ice.

Within minutes Shaun was holding open the door to their room, waving her inside with a very sexy smile that she could not resist. As he let the door shut behind him, she took his hand and tugged him into the centre of the room. Then she began to strip. First her earrings. Then the silver chain from around her neck. Followed by her jacket.

Shaun stood watching her, his tongue circling his lips.

Her dress was next. Lifting it slowly up to reveal her butt, then her stomach and breasts, she did a little wiggle and danced in her heels.

Shaun's eyes widened.

As she seductively slipped the dress over her head, her hips moved in a circle, toward Shaun, away from him.

His hands tightened against his sides. His need pushed out the front of his trousers. He wouldn't be able to wait much longer.

Spinning around on her high heels, she blew him a kiss. Then she unhooked her bra and swung it in the air above her head. Not that Shaun saw that. His focus was entirely on her naked breasts.

'Nikki,' he groaned. His fingers were now fumbling with the buttons on his shirt.

'Shaun.' How was she going to get out of her

nylons without falling over and making an idiot of herself?

Then she was being swung up into his arms and laid on the bed.

Shaun's kiss was deep and long and sent the level of her desire off the scale.

She couldn't tell him to make love to her now because his mouth wasn't leaving hers at all.

At the same time he removed her shoes, then got busy sliding her nylons down over her hips, his hot, firm palms ramping up her need even further. Then he was on her thighs, before going lower to her ankles, and finally the nylons were gone. Then Shaun was tugging his clothes off in haste, no finesse going on. When his erection sprang free, she reached for him, held his penis and rubbed it, up and down.

'Nikki, wait.' He had a condom in his hand.

She took it and slid it over his heat. 'I'm ready.'

Then they were together, as one, bringing each other to the peak. And falling over the precipice into oblivion.

Shaun woke to find himself wrapped around Nikki and smiled happily. Not getting out of bed and leaving her in the middle of the night was a plus. This part of time together was as wonderful as everything else. More so. He felt they'd taken another step forward in their relationship. He hugged her tighter. She was so warm and sexy and good and a load more. What a night they'd shared. A superb dinner at a top-notch restaurant followed by mind-blowing sex more than once at the hotel. He couldn't think of a better way to celebrate his new house. Home.

Nikki hadn't been surprised when he'd told her to pull in to the hotel. It was as though she might've had the same idea. They did appear to think along the same lines about quite a few things, which was good and helped this feel like the beginning of more than a friendship, more like the start of a relationship. If they both were ready for that. He wasn't there yet, but he wasn't averse to the idea anymore.

When Nikki had mentioned her marriage, he'd suspected she wasn't fully over the repercussions. There might be trust issues when it came to believing in a man again. He mightn't have trust problems, but he did struggle to believe he wouldn't again lose someone he loved. Yet Amy had taken the chance and was happy. So why couldn't he give it a try? Because trying wasn't good enough. It had to be for sure or not at all. Though there were never any guarantees about what lay ahead. Knowing it and accepting it were two different aspects of the future he was working towards.

'Morning,' Nikki murmured against his arm lying over her waist.

He brushed a kiss on the back of her neck. 'Morning, Nikki.'

Rolling over, she studied him through sleepy eyes. 'Wow, what a night. I'm glad we stayed right through.'

'I'm not arguing.' He grinned. He hadn't woken this relaxed and in tune with himself in ages. 'Feel like breakfast in bed?' Suddenly he was starving, and for the first time since they'd come to this room, it was for food and not Nikki.

'Absolutely. Though I need a long soak in the shower first.'

'How about we order what we want for half an hour away and then soap each other off?'

Her eyes widened as she grinned. 'Better make that an hour. Sharing a shower might lead to complications. Good ones,' she added with a wicked twist to her grin.

'It's a deal.' He got out of bed to find a menu. He could do sex followed by breakfast. Not a problem. In fact, there wasn't a lot that was a problem with Nikki.

'Have you got any plans for the rest of the day?' Nikki asked when they were finally dressing to leave the hotel.

He paused. Yes, he was going to see his family and tell them the good news. Did he invite Nikki along to meet them? No, she might think he was getting too involved with her, which was the last thing he wanted right now, even if it might be true. Sharing his monumental news with the family was not the same as watching the kids play soccer. 'I'm catching up with my brother and his family. And Mum and Dad.'

'Haven't you told them your news?'

'No. I got sidetracked.' He grinned at her. 'When I left the lawyer, I just had to tell you, and then—well, you know how the night unfolded.'

'I can't deny that.' She slipped her feet into those high heels that turned him on. 'You need to tell your family. They'll be thrilled.'

'They will. What about you? What are you going to do today?'

'I'm catching up with my friend, Molly, and then might drop in on my brother and his family.'

Stepping closer, he wound his arms around her waist. 'Nikki, I have had the most amazing time with you. I'm not walking away from that. We get on brilliantly.'

'But?'

'We haven't known each other very long, and I am not one to rush into things.' Not anymore. He'd done great so far with his plans to settle down here, but if he was going for a permanent relationship, then he had to know it was for real, not something he'd wake up to regret one day. 'I do want to spend more time with you. And with my family. I've missed a lot of time with them and am loving getting to know my nephews better.' He'd invited her to join his family for soccer before it had been cancelled a couple of weeks back. Did she hope he'd ask her along today? 'I would like you to meet my family at some point. I just don't want everyone to read too much into it. Me having bought a house might have them all wondering what else I'm up to.'

A wry smile came his way. 'I'm sorry. It's been an amazing time, and I don't want it to stop. But you're right. We do have separate lives outside this room.'

'We do, and we'll have more great times together.' That wasn't telling her he was looking at a future together, more that they'd see how everything went between them over the coming weeks and months. 'What I mean is that we—'

Her finger touched his lips. 'Stop, Shaun. I get it. I really do. I got carried away and didn't think past leaving the hotel. I am not one of those women who goes home and waits for her phone to ring with someone asking her to join them for the day.'

He couldn't help it. He laughed. 'You honestly think I thought that? You sitting around waiting for other people to bring your life to light? I don't think so.'

'Phew.' Nikki smiled, a little too tightly for his liking. 'Let's get cracking. I'm meeting Molly for coffee soon.'

Nikki was wonderful and becoming more important as the days went by. He wasn't ready to admit that to her, though, or even to himself most of the time. It was too soon. He'd bought a house, and work was going well. Neither had the itch to move on raised its head, which was a positive sign. Everything was working out, but finding a woman he could fall in love with was not to be rushed. Of course, he wanted to love and be loved again. But since meeting Nikki, whenever he thought about love and kids, he got scared. It would be too easy to be hurt if she didn't reciprocate. If she did and it still went wrong, she'd get hurt too, and she'd already been through a nasty divorce. Why was life so darned difficult?

Nikki ran her fingers through her hair in a vain attempt to not look like she'd spent most of the night being active in bed. It was pointless. They had no bags, no overnight gear. The reception staff would know exactly why they'd spent the night in the hotel. Did it matter?

She glanced at Shaun as the lift dropped to the ground floor. No, it didn't. She'd had an amazing night, and so what if other people knew? They didn't know her, weren't about to tell her friends. No, it was fine.

So was Shaun. Despite how he'd suddenly backed away when she'd asked about his plans for the rest of the day. He was right to point out they had lives beyond here that didn't involve them together, and he had told her what he was going to be doing. It was a reminder that they weren't a couple, and that she needed to keep protecting herself.

If only the thought didn't fill her with sadness. For the first time since Brett left, she'd begun to believe there might be a future for her that involved love and family. All because she'd met Shaun. It was still possible, just not this week. She shook her head. She really was rushing in with her eyes wide shut. There was so much she didn't know about this man setting her alight in ways that she'd forgotten were possible. 'Who's the oldest? You or your brother?'

'Me. By eighteen months.'

'That's close in age. Did you get on well or fight all the time?'

'Fought like tigers until we hit the teens, then became best buddies.' Shaun was staring at her. 'Why are you asking?'

Be honest. 'Because I know so little about you other than you're a superb doctor.'

'Only a doctor?' He grinned.

'You're not bad at walking up hills either.' She returned his grin, feeling better by the second.

'Seems I need more practice in certain fields.'

The lift bumped to a halt, and the doors began sliding open. An elderly couple rushed in as though afraid the lift would start moving before the doors closed.

Nikki gave Shaun a sexy wink. At least, she

hoped it was sexy. 'Happy to help sometime.' She wasn't rushing him. She did need to look out for herself.

'I'm sure we can come up with something as entertaining as last night,' he said quiet enough so only she heard.

She blushed. That gravelly voice raised a myriad of memories about the entertainment he was alluding too. Heck, she didn't do blushing. That was for teenagers, not thirty-four-year-old medical specialists. Nudging Shaun with her elbow, she said, 'Get out of here.'

'Can I wait till the lift reaches the lobby?'

Did they have time to go back to the room for another round before checking out? She glanced at Shaun, and he shook his head.

'Afraid not.' His smile hit her in the gut, and she gasped.

This was getting out of hand, and while she was enjoying it, she had to pull the brakes on. They couldn't get too close too soon. It wouldn't be great to have her heart broken again.

CHAPTER NINE

'HOW IS IT that we're nearly always on the same shift?' Shaun commented to Nikki over coffee during a brief lull on Tuesday morning. 'We've hardly done any night or late afternoon ones either.'

'Careful or Paul will put you on nights for the next two months.' Nikki smirked. 'As for me, I did twelve weeks of late shifts when one of the doctors left suddenly, so I'm more than happy with what I'm doing.'

'That must've been exhausting.'

'It was, but I got used to it.' One plus to not having family to worry about or even a dog. 'According to the roster, we're both on late shift next week.' Part of her was pleased she'd still be working with Shaun. Another part worried she was getting too comfortable around him despite wanting to let go of her trust issues. But they worked well together, and frankly, that was good for the patients and other staff.

Michaela came into the tearoom and sat down. 'How was your weekend, Nikki? Go walking?'

'No, didn't get the boots on once. Kept pretty busy, though.' She wasn't looking at Shaun in case that annoying blush returned. Michaela wasn't stupid and would know straight away something was up if it did.

'Shaun?' Michaela asked.

'Spent time with the family, played soccer with the nephews in their backyard before filling them with burgers and chips and getting into trouble with their mum. What about you?'

'Not a lot. We were both tired after a busy week. My husband's a radiologist at the private hospital,' she told Shaun.

Georgie appeared in the doorway. 'Nikki, you're needed. A chopper's about to land with a woman on board who fell off the chairlift on Mount Arthur.'

'Coming.' Forget coffee and the banana muffin she hadn't managed to take a bite from yet. Welcome to their world. 'Anything about the injuries?'

'Suspected broken back,' Georgie informed her.

'Right.' Instantly her mind brought up what she had to do for her patient. It wasn't going to be fun. 'How does someone manage to fall out of a chairlift?'

'By fooling around? Or if the person securing

the bar before they left the hut didn't do it correctly.' Shaun was right beside her. 'Though I thought the method was supposedly infallible.'

Nikki considered who to call to come to see the woman apart from Radiology. Hopefully Charlie was on duty. He was a superb neurosurgeon. 'How long before touchdown, Georgie?'

'Any minute. Sarah's gone up with Cameron to collect the woman, who's conscious, in pain, and can't feel her feet. The emergency doctor on board has got her fixed so she can't move.' Georgie was babbling, which was unlike her.

'You okay?' Nikki asked quietly.

'My best friend broke her back when she was fourteen. Hasn't walked since,' she replied in a strained voice.

Nikki wrapped her arm around Georgie's shoulders. 'You work with other patients, and Cameron can stay on this case. Unless you want to be there, that is.'

Georgie shook her head. 'Not really. It's the one situation I still struggle with. I was with Tracey when it happened, and I still haven't got all those images out of my head.'

'I'm not surprised.' She dropped her arm. 'Some things never leave us, do they?'

'Seems not. Thanks, Nikki.'

For what? She was only doing what she'd want if faced with a similar situation. 'No problem.'

'You're very understanding,' Shaun muttered

as they made their way into the emergency cubicle where their patient would be brought.

'Of course I am,' she snapped. Then felt contrite. 'Sorry. But I know what it's like being reminded of that day I grabbed Jordie from in front of the car, and that was nothing compared to seeing a friend lose her ability to ever walk again.'

'You know because you've been there, faced something horrific.' A shadow was forming in his eyes, as though he also knew was it was like.

'You have too.' Would he say anything about that?

Shaun straightened abruptly and changed the subject. 'Want me to phone Radiology?'

Okay, don't go there. 'Yes, please.' It was starting to irk that he wouldn't talk about the day he had to bring his friend down in the plane. Maybe he never talked about what was important to him, might never open up to her about himself even if they did spend more time together. If so, then she had to keep him at arm's length too. An equal footing, which didn't bode well. So much for getting closer. They weren't. She went to scrub up and prepare for the woman, all the time wondering how Shaun had dealt with the aftermath of that horrendous time he'd gone through.

'Radiology's gearing up for our patient, and someone will be here shortly.' Shaun was back. He looked around. 'Where is this woman?'

'Patience, man.' Nikki said. It was like tiptoeing around on eggshells waiting for someone who was seriously injured to arrive. All ready to go and no one to work on.

'Me? Patient? Not happening.'

Said the man she'd seen to be very patient in tricky situations with people in agony. 'Yeah, right.'

The lift doors slid open. Two men in rescue orange overalls pulled a trolley into the department, followed by Sarah and Cameron.

'Here we go,' Nikki said and crossed over to join them. 'Hello, everyone. How far did our patient fall?'

'About twenty metres is the estimate,' answered the doctor from the helicopter. 'She landed on rocks. She's in and out of consciousness and has lost all feeling from her ankles down.'

Nikki winced. That wasn't good. 'Who is she?'

'Angela Dane, twenty-four, champion skier.'

She recognised the name. 'Let's hope this isn't as serious as it seems.'

'I imagine we'll have another sparring match with the media once this gets out,' Shaun said.

Her shoulders drooped. Hauling them back in place again, she said, 'We'll deal with that later. In here.' She indicated the room they were using. 'Cameron, I want you to stay. Sarah, too. What meds have you given Angela?' she asked the doctor.

He named the painkillers and handed her the

notes he'd written on the way in. 'All here. If there's nothing more you need, we've got to get on our way. There's another woman waiting to be brought in who was in the same chairlift. They're friends and were leaning over the bar looking at some skiers when the lock holding the bar in place gave way. The other woman appears to have got off lightly, possible fractured arm and light concussion. As the second chopper is out on another recovery, we're going back to Mount Arthur for her.'

'See you in a bit.' Nikki was already focusing on Angela, who'd opened her eyes. 'Hello, Angela. You're in hospital. I'm Nikki, an emergency doctor.' She named the rest of the team, but whether Angela took it all in, she wasn't sure.

'I can't feel my feet,' the woman murmured. 'This can't be real. I'm a professional skier. I need my feet.' So she was aware of what was going on around her.

'Angela, I've been told that, but I'd like to check myself.'

'Good. Two opinions are better than one.'

Not if they're the same bad one. Nikki lifted away the blanket covering Angela. 'Tell me if you feel anything on your soles.'

As she pressed her fingertips against one of Angela's heels, then toes and inner foot, the silence was heavy, and upsetting. 'This foot?' The same result. 'What about your ankles?' Again, no reaction. Nikki didn't get any reaction until she touched Angela's knees.

'Yes, I can feel that. Try my feet again.'

Nikki obliged, knowing the result would be the same as before. 'Right, the first thing to be done is have your spine X-rayed. Are you in any pain?' She'd had analgesics, but Nikki needed to know what Angela was feeling now.

'My head hurts. My right arm is agony to move. My back's sore and hurts a lot when I move. But I can't move because the doctor made sure I couldn't.'

'That's so you don't do any more damage while we find out what injuries you have sustained.'

Shaun was examining Angela's elbow and lower arm. 'Multiple fractures here. Did you land on your right side, Angela?'

'Think it was my back, and my arm was under me.'

'That would explain both areas of injuries,' Shaun said.

'There's a deep gouge on her right hip,' Sarah told them.

'Go with her to Radiology, Cameron. We also need an EMI done.' Nikki picked up the phone to call Radiology.

Shaun and Sarah rechecked that Angela couldn't move at all, while Cameron continued monitoring BP, temperature, pulse and more. At one point Shaun looked up and met Nikki's eye.

His face was grim. It wasn't looking good. Angela's competitive days were more than likely over.

Nikki's hand tightened around the phone as she talked to the specialist on the other end. She was supposed to be used to dealing with cases like this, but it didn't matter how often she saw a patient with horrific injuries. It never got any easier. From the look in Shaun's face, it didn't for him either. It didn't for any of them.

'Nikki, wait,' Shaun called after her as she left the department at the end of shift. 'I'll walk out with you.' There were bound to be reporters demanding to know what had happened to Angela Dane. Not so much her friend, who only skied for pleasure. No wonder he hardly ever read or listened to the news these days. It was more often than not one-sided, and exaggerated to boot.

Nikki had a grim smile on her face. 'You're going to get a reputation for always being at my side when the going gets rough.'

Yep, and he found it didn't bother him as much as it once would've. 'Too right I am.' He hoped his smile was a lot more relaxed than hers. 'To hell with journalists. We're doctors here to help people, not to indulge in too much talk.'

Nikki huffed out a breath. 'Did you drive to work? Because I walked, and don't feel like being followed through the park on my way home.'

'It's your lucky day. Why not go out the side door?'

'Because it rarely works when it comes to avoiding the reporters, and besides, I need to stare them down and ignore what they ask. There's no avoiding them, so I might as well get on with whatever they throw my way.'

Go, Nikki. 'Of course, they may not have heard about Angela Dane's accident.'

'You're kidding, right? Not only will they have heard she's injured, but they'll know that the chairlift failed. Even if that's an exaggeration, they'll know something went wrong with it. I wouldn't like to be the poor people on the ski field working the chairlifts right now. Though I suppose they stopped using them from the moment the women fell.'

'You're right. There'll be an enquiry.' Shaun suddenly realised he was holding Nikki's elbow. When had he done that? She wasn't pulling away. Because she needed his support? Or because, like him, she hadn't realised what he was doing? Whichever, he wasn't letting go while she was comfortable with his action. He liked being there for her, even though she didn't need his support. She was strong and could stare down anyone who got in her face. But that didn't mean he wasn't watching her back.

The hospital foyer was no different to most days, people coming and going, some looking stressed, others carrying bunches of flowers and talking non-stop to their companions.

'So far so good,' Nikki said.

As they walked outside and headed to his car, reporters began shouting questions at them, and he felt Nikki take a deep breath. 'Ignore them.'

'I intend to.'

'Shaun, are you all right?' a female reporter called.

Afraid the woman would mention Liam's story, he moved faster. It was not how he wanted Nikki to learn what had happened. 'Let's get out of here.'

She upped her pace. 'I'm with you all the way.'

The time was fast approaching when he'd have to talk to Nikki about his past. He didn't wanted her to hear about it from anyone else, but telling her wouldn't be easy. He'd be showing her how vulnerable he'd been, and maybe still was.

When they reached his SUV, she said, 'Thanks for that. I'd have stopped to say I couldn't tell them a thing, which would've got me nowhere.'

'Feel like going for a drink to let off steam?'

Finally a beautiful light-up-his-world smile came his way. 'Sounds perfect.' Then she got in his vehicle and buckled herself in. 'Where should we go?'

'There's great little bar in the centre of the city. It's quiet, and I doubt anyone will find us there.'

'Sounds ideal.'

Unless she began asking why that reporter knew him. Of course all she had to do was go online, and she'd soon learn what had happened. But was she that kind of person? Or would she wait until he told her his story? If he didn't tell her without prompting, what did that say about him, or where they were at? He had no idea at the moment, only understood he was beginning to fall for her, and the time was coming when he'd have to front up about his fears. In the meantime, he'd continue to try to go slowly, saviour the good moments. Except going slow wasn't working. He couldn't get enough of her, which was scaring the pants off him. Laughter tripped over his lips.

'Want to share the joke?'

Hell no. Then again, why not? 'I was thinking how quickly you manage to get me to remove my pants at times.'

'That's all up to me, is it?'

He laughed again. She knew how to make him relax and put aside the fears he carried. 'If you weren't with me, it wouldn't be happening.'

'Glad to hear it.' She grinned, looking relaxed again.

They were a good team, both at work and away from the department.

Later, after an early dinner, they went back to Nikki's and proved just that.

* * *

As soon as she finished work on Friday, Nikki headed straight to her favourite clothing shop that happened to be owned by Paul's wife. Shaun was taking her out to dinner again, and she wanted to look as good as she could. So much for backing off. She couldn't stay clear of him.

'Hello, Nikki. I haven't seen you in here in ages, so you must have a hot date lined up. Who's the lucky man?' asked Mallory when she walked into the shop. 'Not Shaun Elliott by any chance?'

'You might be right.' Nikki laughed. Strange how she no longer wanted to keep quiet among her friends about the fact they were dating. How he'd feel about that was anyone's guess, but for once, she was comfortable with a relationship and wasn't going to hide it.

'Awesome. Everyone liked him at the dinner. Now, what are you looking for?'

'We're going to dinner, and I want to look a bit swish.' If that was possible. Hopefully she could turn out all right with a bit of help from Mallory.

'Any particular colour in mind? Style?'

'Not black or white. Fitting without showing the bumps.'

'What bumps? You've got a lovely figure.' Mallory was already at a rack of evening dresses and lifting a red dress off the rail. 'What do you think of this?'

Immediately she fell in love with it. The satin

midi frock with a deep vee neckline was sleeveless. A wide waist band flowed into the floating skirt. 'Beautiful.' It had better fit perfectly or she'd be gutted. Since when did she get in such a fuss about an evening dress? Since she'd fallen for Shaun, that's when.

'Come on. Let's get you trying it on.' Mallory led the way to a fitting room. 'I can't wait to see you wearing it.'

'You're certain it'll fit, aren't you?'

'I know my job, Nikki, so don't prove me wrong.'

Within minutes Nikki was strolling around feeling like she'd touched down in Paradise. 'It's beautiful.' Hadn't she already said that?

'It's a perfect fit.' Mallory got serious. 'Right, shoes next. You need a jacket too as it won't be warm tonight. Winter hasn't let its grip go yet.'

When Nikki walked out of the shop nearly an hour later, she was smiling so hard it almost hurt. When had she spent so much on clothes for one evening? Never was the answer.

Then Shaun walked in her front door and nearly tripped over his feet when he saw her. She knew it was worth every single cent.

'You look stunning. Wow. I mean—' He shoved his fingers through his hair, mussing it a little. 'I'm behaving like a horny teen, but seriously.'

She laughed. He knew how to make her feel

good about herself. 'Seriously nothing. I felt like sprucing up a little.' Sometimes she did need to know she was attractive to a man. After Brett, she'd often doubted it, but tonight she'd made the grade.

'Hey, come here, my girl. You are beautiful—even dressed in scrubs.' Shaun kissed her lightly. 'I mean it.'

My girl? She'd take that as a positive. But as for the scrubs scenario, 'You might be going a bit far there.'

'Me? Never. Right, are you ready? We should hit the road or else we might not make dinner, and I don't really want to get you out of that dress yet.'

Picking up the small evening bag she'd added to her purchases, she grinned. 'Ready as I'll ever be.'

'Let's go.' There was a bounce in his step as they walked out to his SUV.

The bounce didn't dim all evening. Or all night for that matter.

Only in the morning when Nikki's alarm went off did Shaun suddenly turn serious. 'What time is it?'

'Seven thirty. I've got a hair appointment at ten.'

Shaun leapt out of bed. 'I'm meant to be meeting the kids at their soccer game at nine thirty, and it's out at Lyttelton. Before then, I have to pick up a present for my sister-in-law, Sandy. It's her birthday.'

'Slow down. You've got plenty of time.' What was the panic? Two hours was enough to do all that.

'You're right. I have.' He leaned across the bed and kissed her lightly. 'But I should go home and get tidied up first.'

'Fair enough. Will we catch up later?'

'Not today I'm afraid. I'm due at Sandy's birthday dinner at my brother's. But how about we go for a hike tomorrow? Try one around Lyttelton?'

'Sounds good to me.'

'I'll call later to arrange a pick-up time.'

'How about I drive up for a change?' She hadn't been inside where he currently lived. Then again, she had seen where he was moving to, so he wasn't keeping her at arm's length. It rubbed her up the wrong way whenever he kept things to himself now.

'Because I like driving.' He gave her a self-mocking smile. 'It's the male side of my personality looking out for you.'

'Get out of here. See you tomorrow.' She didn't want him to leave, but that was the nature of this relationship. They did spend more time together than she'd have believed a couple of weeks ago, and she was loving it, so she let it go for now.

'Bye.' Shaun disappeared out of the bedroom. Moments later, the front door banged shut.

Nikki pinched herself to make sure he really had been here and they'd had incredible sex more than once. No wonder she felt tired and ached in places. She hadn't had so much exercise in forever. She laughed. So where to from here? More sex for one. More walks and dinners. Dating was a lot of fun. For the first time since she'd found herself single again, she was making the most of every moment. Especially the ones spent with Shaun. She was happy when not querying everything he said and did, and not waiting for the clang when he said enough was enough and he was off to find someone more obliging and loving.

Shaun could still do that.

Yes, he might. Yet she wanted to believe he wouldn't. Probably setting herself up for a big fall, but having decided to start putting herself out there in an attempt to find true love, she wasn't backing off without good reason.

Throwing the bedcovers aside, she leapt out of bed and went to have a long, hot shower to ease the aches before getting ready to go to the hairdresser. Maybe she could ask for a different style. She'd kept her hair long and straight for years and suddenly felt like a change. A bit like that dress she bought yesterday. It'd been stunning and more revealing than her norm, and she'd enjoyed every moment wearing it. Especially the gleam it brought to Shaun's eyes. Oh yes. Thinking about him made her grin. Except she really had no idea what was going on with both of them.

Standing in the driveway of his house, Shaun tossed the keys to the front door in the air and caught them again. Toss, catch. Toss, catch. The previous owners had moved out early and were happy for him to have the keys before the take-over date. He'd been coming around here every day with the intention of making decisions about colour schemes for when it came to redecorating and what sort of furniture he'd like. He hadn't asked anyone to come with him to help with those decisions. Not even Nikki. They were choices he had to make himself because he was the one going to live here. As in he now really and truly owned a house in Christchurch where his family were. Life couldn't get much better.

It was the biggest decision he's made so far. What next? Yes, well, he was having a wonderful time dating Nikki. More than wonderful. She was everything he could wish for and more. Going out to dinner had been special, like every date they went on. As for that incredible dress she wore to dinner—it had lit up her eyes and made her look drop-dead gorgeous, out of this world. Followed by making out in her bed and staying through-out the night. Walking in the hills on Sunday had been a bonus as they'd gone for a meal in Lyttel-ton afterwards. Over the past week, they'd had another, less upmarket, meal together, and he'd stopped over at her place after.

Did this mean he was getting serious about where they were going with their relationship? He *was* falling for Nikki. She had his heart in her hand, but he was not prepared to accept that completely. There were moments when he had to step away and take a deep breath because he was still worried that he didn't deserve being happy when Liam couldn't. He still hadn't told Nikki about how he'd lost Liam and hence Amy. At times it still felt raw, though less since meeting Nikki. Did that mean she could wipe away his fears and become a permanent part of his life? He hoped so, and would work hard to make it possible.

Unfortunately he didn't know how Nikki felt about them. Was she happy with things as they were? Or was she wanting more, like the whole relationship thing? If she didn't, then he was setting himself up for more heartache. And he wasn't sure he could take that again.

'Hi there. Are you our new neighbour?' A middle-aged guy stood at the end of the driveway. 'I've seen you a couple of times over the past few days so figured you must be. I'm Colin.'

'Hey, Colin. I'm Shaun Elliott, and yes, your new neighbour.' He shook Colin's extended hand. 'I haven't moved in yet. Still haven't bought any furniture.' But he was heading to the furniture store shortly to start on selecting what he liked.

He had given notice on the flat he was renting and was ready to move in once he had some furniture.

'It's always a hassle shifting house. Getting everything put in the right place and unpacking the millions of boxes of stuff you never use.'

Shaun laughed. 'I come very light. Very few cartons and at the moment no furniture.' Furnished flats had been his way since breaking up with Amy, and he wasn't a hoarder of junk.

'Obviously you don't have a wife then.'

No laugh this time. 'No, I don't.'

Colin looked contrite. 'I'll leave you to it. If you want a hand with anything like moving furniture when you get some, give me a shout. We're on your left.'

'Thanks. I will.' Only if to get back onside with the man. It didn't pay to upset neighbours. You never knew when you might need them. 'When I move in, come over and have a beer with me.'

Colin looked relieved. 'Sure will. See you around.'

Inside Shaun wandered from room to room, trying to soak up the feeling of being on track, except it wasn't happening. It was as though what Colin said had burst his bubble. Asking about a wife shouldn't tip everything askew in his mind. But he was off centre now. This was his permanent home. But looking around the bare lounge, he suddenly felt at a loss over how to cope. He'd never done anything like this on his own. Making decisions about colour schemes and furniture to suit himself was alien, and while it should have been exciting, he was confused.

Is that how he'd react if he did fall in love with Nikki? Be happy one day, messed up and out of it the next? Nikki, Nikki. She filled his mind so often it should be thrilling, except right now it was worrying.

Calm down. Take your time. Start with getting the house sorted before anything else.

He looked around, half expecting to see Liam in the doorway.

Of course he wasn't there. But those words remained. They were right. He had to get a grip and work his way through everything that needed doing piece by piece, not try to do it all at once. Easy said. Darn sight harder to do.

His phone rang. Nikki. To answer or not? Toughen up. 'Hey, how's things?'

'Can't complain. Wondered if you'd like to drop in for dinner later on? I've put together a venison casserole.'

'Venison, eh? You're not into hunting by any chance?'

'No way. But Ross is. My brother,' she added.

'Yes, you've mentioned him.' Often. They appeared to be close, unlike their parents. What had it been like to never settle in one place and be able to make permanent friends? Worse than the last years he'd spent on the move, he'd bet. Something to remember about Nikki. He did not want to be one of those people who upended her world to satisfy his own needs as her father had. That made the thought to take his time getting settled before deepening their relationship more important. So did he accept her invitation? It wasn't out of the blue. They were friends. In other words, yes, despite the tightness in his belly.

'Hello? You still there?'

'Sorry. I got sidetracked. Dinner would be great, venison being one of my favourite meats. I'll bring some wine.' Red would go well. 'But I might be a bit late as I'm going furniture shopping first.'

'Want some help with that? I love trying out lounge suites.' Her laugh nudged his mood upwards.

'Is there no stopping you? I'm heading to Furniture Central. See you there.'

Walking into the massive furniture store, he hesitated. This wasn't going to be easy. The range of lounge suites alone was mind-boggling. Where to start?

'There you are.' Nikki appeared in front of him.

'Where am I going to start?'

'What's most important to you? The lounge, kitchen dining room or your bedroom? Focus on one, and then everything else will fall into place.'

He shrugged. Made sense—if he knew which was the most important. 'My bedroom.' Then he'd have somewhere to sleep and could move in sooner than later. Hopefully selecting a bed would be straightforward compared with lounge furniture.

Nikki slid her arm through his. 'You look lost.'

'A little.' There were beds in all directions and headboards and bedside tables with every single one. 'I want a super king-size bed, and not one that you can raise the mattress.' Surely that would narrow the options a little.

Nikki wandered around for a few minutes. 'Guess we can't try them out,' she said, grinning.

The tension was back, harder than before. This wasn't how he wanted to do this. The furniture was for him. But he had agreed to Nikki coming along, so he'd have to suck it up. He could. He would.

'Shaun? Problem?' The grin had disappeared.

'I'm fine.'

'No, you're shutting down on me.'

True. 'You think?'

'I know.'

Deep breath. 'Sorry. Come on, let's find me a bed.'

Thirty minutes later, Shaun sighed with relief. He'd chosen a bed and bedside tables. 'One room done.'

'What's next?'

'Lounge suite, or maybe two reclining chairs. Preferably leather.'

As he followed Nikki he looked around the huge area and began to feel overwhelmed. This was getting serious. He'd bought a house and been thrilled, but choosing furniture made everything more real. This was permanent. It was going to be all right. Was it though?

For the first time since he'd arrived in Christchurch, the familiar itch was beginning to make itself felt deep in his gut, reminding him he couldn't stay in one place for long. Soon he'd have to move on.

'What colour do you prefer?' Nikki again.

He could do this. He was not moving away. He was not. 'Dark green.'

'Over there.'

He strode in the direction she pointed, his back tight, his gut getting in a tizz. *I am staying.* The reclining chairs were exactly what he liked. He sat down on one and pulled the lever to make it recline. Yes, it was comfortable, but he wasn't. This was serious, being here and looking to buy everything to make his life right, to make his house a home with Nikki watching.

Sitting up abruptly, Shaun got back on his feet and began walking away. This was wrong. He couldn't settle down. Not yet. Maybe never.

'What's wrong?' Nikki asked.

'I think I'll leave the rest for another day. I'll

pay for the bedroom furniture now and organise a delivery time, then go.' He *was* staying, wasn't moving away. But first he was getting out of here.

To go to Nikki's for dinner. Oh hell. He couldn't. He didn't trust himself to remain calm, and not to tell her everything going on in his mind.

'Still on for dinner? Nikki asked.

He couldn't let her down. That wasn't right when she'd come here to help him with decisions about furniture. He hadn't asked her to. Damn it. He was between a rock and a hard place. Just what he'd spent years avoiding. 'I'll be right behind you.'

CHAPTER TEN

SHAUN SAT OPPOSITE Nikki at the table, each with a plate of casserole and rice in front of them. He'd hardly spoken since he'd got here, and he knew she was fed up about something. 'What's going on, Nikki?'

'Nothing.'

His mood had gone downhill fast in the furniture store as it sank in what he was doing. This was a permanent move, one he wanted more than anything, but suddenly reality had hit, making him feel scared. Now he longed to know what Nikki was thinking. 'Try again, Nikki.'

'Are you regretting buying the house by any chance?'

'Not at all.'

'You'd have preferred I hadn't joined you looking for furniture? Your mood changed big-time there.'

'No, I appreciated your help.' He really did.

'Then tell me what's bugging you. Is your past hindering you?'

Leaning back, he studied her, wondering where this was going. Did she know what had happened? Had Paul told her? He'd better not have. It was his to tell, no one else's.

'What?' she demanded. He hadn't been forthcoming about Liam or his marriage, and now he regretted that. He also wished she'd talked more about her past. He hadn't asked, knowing how hard it could be to do. But what if Nikki didn't trust him enough to share her story? His heart plummeted. That would break him.

'Nikki, neither of us have talked about our pasts. I know little about your marriage and how you feel about getting involved with another man. Do you trust men? Me?'

The fork she'd been holding dropped onto her plate with a clang. 'You want to know that now? What's it got to do with your mood swing?'

'I'm finding a few obstacles as I make this a permanent move, but don't ever doubt that I am here for good.' She still wasn't giving of herself.

'Trying to convince me or yourself?'

He sat upright. 'How about answering my question? I'd really like to know more about what makes you tick, Nikki.' So far she'd seemed happy to share her time with him, but it now seemed not who she really was. Her explanation about losing her baby and husband had been very brief, with little about how she'd coped and what she felt going forward. Did she even want another relationship? He had no idea.

'Sounds familiar,' she snapped. 'I know about how you brought down that Cessna with your friend on board. Why haven't you talked to me about that? About how it's affected you? I presume that's why you haven't been able to settle in one place since it happened.'

He said nothing.

Nikki drew a breath as she waited, hoping against hope he'd talk to her. He was right though. She hadn't talked about Brett and how broken she'd been over losing him and their baby for fear Shaun would think she was too needy and run for cover. She'd spent the intervening years since Brett left getting back on her feet, afraid of losing her way. She did want a second chance at love but had been afraid she didn't deserve it. If Brett could walk away so easily, so could the next man she gave her heart to. But she had to try. This was too important to give up on. Obviously Shaun wasn't about to open up, so she continued. 'Don't you trust me to understand how the loss of your friend would've affected you?'

Shaun shook his head, sadness filling his eyes. 'I could ask you the same question regarding your marriage, and about losing your baby, but I haven't because I hoped you'd tell me without prompting. Yes, I do understand how that feels.' Standing up, he looked at her with sorrow. 'I guess neither of us is ready to talk about ourselves. Which means neither of us is ready to go any further with this.' Then he walked out of the room to the front door, leaving her decimated.

She had no answer to that, because he was right. They weren't ready. But neither could they get there if he was gone.

He'd blown it. Shaun groaned as he got into the SUV. He should've kept a lid on his emotions, but they were roiling around his body, getting him into a tight knot that he couldn't find a way to unravel. Nikki had come to mean so much to him, yet he still couldn't tell her. He couldn't show her how vulnerable he felt after losing the two people he'd loved so much.

How long had she known about the Cessna incident? She'd probably always known. With major headlines on the TV and internet news coverage here and overseas, it would've been hard not to. To be fair, she understood too well what that was like and how it played with your head. She never talked about saving Jordie, though they had both admitted struggling to cope with the day in the department when those people were hit by the bus. He hadn't explained why he felt that way, nor had Nikki mentioned her story, presumably because he'd told a reporter he knew about it.

He banged his hand on the steering wheel.

What a mess. So much for thinking he was on track with his plans for the future. But he was. So why had spending time in the house looking around thrown him off centre? The house was right for him. Was that the problem? For him, and not for anyone else to join him? When the neighbour mentioned a wife, he'd felt a weight come down on him. And when Nikki turned up at the furniture shop all bubbly and happy, nothing at all felt right.

Pressing the button to start the engine, he glanced towards Nikki's front door. She stood in the doorway, highlighted by the lights behind her long hair falling over her shoulders and her tight stance, no longer bubbly and happy. Neither was he. But this had to be a blip, nothing major to upset his determination to stay here. Because he was staying, no matter what.

Nikki watched Shaun accelerate away. Despite his change in demeanour at the furniture shop, he'd accepted her invitation for a meal and even said he'd bring wine. When he hadn't, she'd got out one of hers. No problem. Neither of them had finished their meal, had been merely pushing it around their plates with a fork. Nor had the wine been touched. Was this the end of what they'd had? It felt like it.

'What the heck is your problem, Shaun?' she asked as his taillights disappeared round the corner. 'Why the mood change?' He'd been so thrilled to have bought the house, yet something had upset him. After going inside, she slammed the door shut and locked it before heading to the kitchen to drink her wine.

'Shaun Elliott, you owe me an explanation for walking away.' From the moment he'd put in an offer on that house, he'd been ecstatic and on tenterhooks until the deal was finalised. Now it seemed he'd come crashing down off the high. Did he have regrets about buying it? He'd said he was home for good. Was that it? He didn't want to stay after all?

It was the one thing she'd feared when she started falling for him. She couldn't stand the thought he'd move away, or want to keep moving time after time, yet she'd let him into her heart anyway. Because she couldn't stop him. She was ready to take a chance on love, all because she'd met Shaun. He'd been the tipping point, and she didn't regret it until tonight. She hadn't done anything wrong that she could see, and she thought she knew him well enough to think he'd have told her otherwise. But then, she wasn't great at understanding the men she came to care about. Look how badly she'd messed up by believing Brett loved her and only her.

You didn't explain how Brett had made you distrustful about loving someone again when he asked. You owe Shaun that as much as he needs to talk to you.

Taking a big sip of wine, she looked for her phone. They had to move beyond this, couldn't give up so easily. She pressed his number.

'Nikki.'

'Hi, Shaun. Are you okay?'

'I'm fine,' he snapped.

Which said to her he wasn't. 'Then why did you leave?'

Silence.

'Shaun, talk to me.'

'I'm pulling over.' A moment later he continued. 'I apologise for my behaviour. It's been a busy day, and I'm exhausted. Just want to get home and curl up for a good sleep.'

Just as well she hadn't put on her new sexy little number, because she didn't believe him, and it would've been demeaning if he'd reacted like she was a nuisance if she came on to him. 'You could've taken the time to tell me what was bothering you.'

'Yes, you're right, I probably should've, but I needed to get away and be on my own.'

That hurt. Big-time. 'I thought we were better than this.'

'Seems we both have problems talking about our pasts. I'll see you at shift changeover tomorrow.' He hung up.

Something was definitely wrong, and now she

was more convinced it was to do with her. If he'd gone off her, all he had to do was say so and not accept her dinner invitation. He could've said he hadn't needed her to help select furniture. Everything had been going well. The nights together in bed, the meals they shared, working alongside each other. But still, she hadn't been very forthcoming about her past either.

Work. Great. How was she going to manage that comfortably if Shaun wasn't talking to her? Guess she'd find out soon enough.

Shaun rolled his shoulders and rubbed his lower back. He was tired beyond reason. He'd barely slept a wink since their argument thinking of Nikki and his house and ticking off that damned list. Why had he even drawn it up in his head? It was always going to lead to disaster.

'Doc, I think I'm going to be sick,' said the eighteen-year-old lying on the bed in front of him.

Shaun grabbed the bowl the nurse had placed on the cabinet. 'Use this.' The guy had been brought in with concussion after falling off a ladder in the storeroom where he worked. 'Vomiting's a normal reaction to hitting your head.'

'I've got this,' Georgie said. 'Paul wants you in emergency cubicle two.'

'I'll be back shortly.' Shaun went to see what was going on in the next cubicle. Except it was

Nikki attending to the patient, not Paul. 'I hear I'm wanted.'

'This is Maria. She suffered severe chest pain while playing golf.'

'Cardiac arrest?'

'Yes. Lucky for her, help was right at the golf club.'

He got down to business, helping Nikki with the patient, not quite sure why he'd been called on.

When a cardiologist arrived, Shaun went back to see his other patient. 'How're you feeling?'

'Better now I've thrown up.'

'We'll keep you here for a couple of hours, and if nothing else goes wrong, you'll be free to head home.' He filled the guy in on what drugs he'd prescribe for the pain. 'Stay away from ladders for a while. Another knock on your head could have serious repercussions.'

'You on for a coffee break?' Georgie asked as they left the cubicle.

'Definitely.' Along with something to eat. He hadn't had more than one piece of toast for breakfast, and now his stomach was complaining.

Nikki was sitting at the table when they entered the staffroom and said, 'Maria's going up to ICU as I speak. She's in a bad way.'

'I'm not surprised. Her readings indicated a major cardiac event. She doesn't know how lucky she was not to arrest.' He poured a coffee from the plunger and went to sit on the opposite side of the table. Directly in line with Nikki's gaze. Damn it. He missed her like he couldn't believe. After her phone call as he drove away the other night, she'd been aloof towards him. He wasn't blaming her. He'd messed up. Would she give him a second chance? She could say what she liked. He'd listen and try to find a way through this mess they'd got into.

'Has Paul mentioned the group dinner next weekend?' Nikki asked, surprising him.

Maybe there was a chance. He shook his head. 'No, but he knows I won't be here.' He was sorry he'd miss getting together with them all. They were fun and friendly and added to his sense of belonging, which right now was headed out the window. All because everything had gone too well and frightened him.

'You're on holiday for the weekend?'

'For five days actually. To Adelaide.'

She pulled a face. 'You never mentioned it. But then, I don't suppose you had to tell me everything you're up to.'

Had, as in the past. He glanced around, but thankfully Georgie was nowhere to be seen. This was getting a little personal. Pain enveloped him. It wasn't what he wanted. He wanted to leap up and pull Nikki into his arms and hold on to her, but that wouldn't be right when he was so unsure of himself. 'Nikki, I'm sorry. I seem to have hit a wall and need to move around it before I know what I'm doing next.'

The mug moved back and forwards in her hands. She watched him closely for a long moment. 'You know you can talk to me anytime you want.'

Surprised, he shook his head. 'Thanks, but I prefer working through my problems by myself.'

Her head jerked up, and her eyes widened with something like anger as she stared at him as though he was a complete stranger to her.

He waited to be blasted with criticism for being selfish. If only he had talked to her about the past when they were getting along. It would've been easier. Now every time he opened his mouth, he seemed to hurt her. Now it was too late. He'd hurt her when he'd been trying hard not to hurt either of them. She wouldn't forgive him for that. She held her heart tight and wasn't giving it away easily. He didn't want Nikki feeling sorry for him, or staying around because she thought he might feel worse if she dumped him.

'Fine.' She stood up, placed her mug in the dishwasher and strode out to the room with a very straight back and long strides.

The message was loud and clear. She was done with him, whether he changed his mind about how he felt or not.

One thing to come out of the days of going over everything countless times was that he had fallen for her. But that wasn't enough. He had to trust himself to stay around, had to believe his heart would be safe with her, had to know hers would be more than safe with him, and at the moment he was a bit wobbly where that was concerned. He couldn't trust himself to see through his plans to settle back here. Since buying the house, it had become clear how much harder it was to let go of the past than he'd thought. So much for thinking he was ready. Obviously he wasn't.

Maybe he should look for a new position in Adelaide while he was there for his sister's wedding.

When he finished his shift, Shaun went directly to his house as he'd had a message saying the store was delivering more furniture in the afternoon. He'd no sooner stepped inside when the sound of a truck backing up the drive had him walking out the front door.

A man hopped out of the passenger side of the delivery truck. 'Hey, mate. I've got a load for Shaun Elliott. That be you?'

'Sure is. What've you got?' He'd been back to the store and chosen more items in the hope it would quieten his concerns about staying. It hadn't worked, but he'd do anything to stick to the plan.

'A lounge suite and a table and chairs. There's more to come tomorrow morning if you're about.'

His house was becoming his home, yet he

didn't feel right about it. Falling out with Nikki had killed a lot of his happiness and hope. Even work didn't feel as comfortable at the moment. Instead he was constantly questioning if he was doing the right thing by staying on.

He'd worked the evening shift when he overheard Kennedy saying his son was sick and he wanted to be with him. It meant he didn't have to rub shoulders with Nikki until he flew out to Adelaide. Time off to go to the wedding had been part of the deal when he signed up with the department. He hadn't mentioned it to Nikki out of habit. Another mistake, but it didn't matter now. She'd learned he was going away, and they weren't spending time together anyway.

'Show us where you want this stuff and we'll get on with the job, and then we can knock off for the day.'

'Come in.' He led the man inside and pointed out the rooms where the furniture was going. 'I'll give you a hand.'

'Thanks, but me and my offsider have got this. Though you could bring in the dining chairs.'

The lighter pieces. He supposed it made sense. These guys were used to hauling furniture around. He wasn't. It didn't take long for the three of them to unload everything. 'I can't even offer you a beer,' Shaun said as they finished up. 'The fridge hasn't arrived.' Along with the freezer and a new dishwasher since the one that had been here wasn't in great condition. Seemed strange they hadn't been delivered when the saleswoman had said they had some in stock. Then again, it didn't really matter. He wasn't living here yet.

'No problem, mate. See you in the morning with the next load.' They were gone, obviously in a hurry for that beer.

Shaun wished he did have a cold beer on hand so he could drink a toast to his house and maybe improve his mood, but knew it would take more than a beer to do that. There was more furniture to decide on, and his few books and other possessions to unpack, which hopefully would make everything feel right again. He imagined his nephews running around the lawn kicking the hell out of their soccer ball and yelling at each other just like he and his brother used to at that age. Kids. He'd always wanted a family. He and Amy talked about it often, coming up with names and how many they might have when they finally got around to it. They'd intended waiting until he'd specialised so he'd be on hand for the kids more, and he didn't want to miss out on too much time with them. Then it all went belly up.

It hurt, but nowhere near as much as usual. He had to believe he was moving on and getting used to the idea of a second chance, yet it wasn't true. He felt lonely and empty, longing for Nikki to be at his side again. But how to overcome this? Anything he said to Nikki could do more damage, not repair the hurt he'd caused. Love could be forgiving and wonderful, and sometimes it couldn't cope with life's atrocities.

Wandering through the house once more, he wondered if he wanted to share it with someone—with Nikki. Living here alone forever was not what he'd hoped for. Nor did he want just anyone here with him. Nikki would be the one if he did take that last step. Not ready. Not by a long way, despite caring about her so much it hurt. They couldn't even have a conversation about their pasts without getting wound up with each other. There was a lot they hadn't talked about. He didn't know how she felt about having children now that she'd lost one. Losing the baby and her husband within weeks of each other had to have cut deep. That man leaving her while she grieved could have well and truly put her off ever wanting to try for a family again.

He had tried asking Nikki about it, and look where that got him. Out in the cold, because he hadn't been able to talk about himself either.

It *was* time to open up about his past, to expose his fears, make himself vulnerable, if he wanted to achieve his dreams.

I'm not ready.

Nikki was in his heart. That didn't mean he was ready to step up and declare his love. Not by a long way. So much for thinking he was moving on. Especially when Nikki might still have issues with her past. She didn't need a man in her life who could wake up one morning and say it was time to move on to a new place and ask her to go with him. She'd made it perfectly clear she was settled and wasn't prepared to go somewhere else to start over with new friends when she obviously had a great circle of pals here already. No doubt for the first time in her life, if he'd understood how moving around as a child had affected her.

It was time to take a step back and think everything through properly. For both their sakes. He did not want to go through the pain he'd known when he lost both Liam and Amy. Nikki didn't need additional pain any more than he did.

He walked outside and around his home. Yes, his home. He'd get there. He had to for his sake if no one else's. But he wasn't taking that final step with Nikki until he was absolutely certain he could last the distance. Just thinking about Liam and Amy had his heart racing and the fear returning.

But he owed Nikki an apology for being blunt yesterday.

Tugging his phone from his pocket, he stared at her number.

He'd let her down.

Which would be worse? To apologise and possibly raise her hopes he wanted to get together again? Or to be honest and tell her he wasn't ready to commit to a relationship?

He slid the phone back into his pocket.

Nikki was still peeved over how Shaun had treated her. So much for thinking they got along well. He hadn't been forthcoming about himself, but she'd thought he'd slowly get over it and talk to her about why he didn't stay in one place for long and why this time he was determined to settle down.

But she was also angry with herself.

One thing that was very clear was she loved him. Not a little but completely. But she also wasn't going to be treated like she didn't matter. Either they were together or they weren't, and he'd gone for the second option. She needed to know why if she was going to be able to move on. *Move on.* The phrase that had haunted her since she lost her baby and then her husband. Yet after only a few weeks with Shaun, here she was thinking she could do it. No doubt she'd been reading too much into their dates and sex. It was no more than a fling, but since she'd finally loosened the knots around her heart, she'd found more to their relationship than was really there.

'Stuff you, Shaun. You've hurt me, and I need to know why.' Shoving her plate aside, she grabbed her laptop and began typing. She'd put off doing this to give him the opportunity to tell her and got nowhere. And yes, she did feel guilty for not talking about how Brett had decimated her with his infidelity. There had been a moment or two when she could've sucked up her fears and got on with explaining why she felt so vulnerable.

Shaun Elliott, NZ.

Ping. His name came up more than once, along with photos of him looking distraught.

Shaun Elliott did all he could to save his friend's life in the skies over Christchurch.

Shaun Elliott, doctor, not a pilot, brought plane down, with dead friend.

Shaun Elliott refuses to talk to media.

On and on it went. Many details about Liam having a cardiac arrest while flying the plane and Shaun being unable to save him. How Shaun worked hard to bring his friend back to his family in one piece. How he hadn't been able to do CPR.

Nikki leaned back in her chair. Sweat broke out on her forehead. Her heart pounded. How did anyone move past that? Shaun definitely hadn't. He'd been caught in an impossible situation. It had been in the news for days. No wonder he'd been short with the reporters on the day the people hit by that bus came into ED. It also explained why he'd had her back the whole time. He definitely understood what it was like to be continuously hounded by the press.

Something they had in common. But she hadn't kept her feelings to herself when with friends. Talking to Molly and others had helped her get through the worst days. Did Shaun talk to his family about what happened that day? She'd listen without butting in every few minutes if he'd let her, but she knew he wouldn't let her anywhere near. It was time to let it all go, if that was possible, and leave it up to Shaun to decide if and when he was going to talk about his past. If she didn't, then she'd only end up bitter and angry with herself.

He hadn't even mentioned that he was going away for a few days at any time they'd been talking about places they liked to visit. Why was he going to Adelaide? Looking into a new job? But he'd bought a house here, had said he was staying, settling down to be near his family.

Her head throbbed with all the questions and no answers. Time to leave it alone. She needed to sleep, having had little last night because once again Shaun had been in her head all night long. Why had she been so stupid to let him into her heart?

Because she'd had no choice. One day she hadn't known him. Less than a week later he was setting her alight with need and a longing for the life she no longer believed possible. Now he was in her heart.

It was time to pull on her big girl pants and look out for herself.

But as she lay in bed waiting for sleep to take over, she couldn't stop thinking about Shaun and how it must've been in that plane that he couldn't fly with his friend dying at his feet. He had mentioned nightmares after the bus accident. Now she understood why he had them. Like hers with the car repeatedly racing towards Jordie and her.

The car that grew bigger and bigger the closer it got until the bonnet was in her face. Then the front was slamming into her legs. Jordie was screaming as they became airborne. Screaming and screaming. Both of them. Slam. Onto the road. Pain. Excruciating.

Nikki jerked awake, sat up fast. Sweat poured down her face. Damn it. When were these nightmares going to stop? Why tonight when she hadn't dealt with anything traumatic in the department? Other than Shaun's cold shoulder, and that shouldn't have brought on the nightmare.

Her heart was thumping, making her ribs ache. Her head felt full of air. Damn you, Shaun. He could take the blame since he'd messed up her heart. But she had to take the guilt she carried about not telling him about herself and explaining why she found it hard to talk about her vulnerability.

Climbing out of bed, she pulled on her thick bathrobe and went to make a cup of tea. And thought more about their last conversation here. He hadn't been forthcoming. But neither had she, instead turning it back on him. She hated exposing her pain over losing her baby, and then Brett, hated admitting how wrong she'd been about her ex. Talking about it only brought all the anger and hurt and disappointment roaring back, making her vulnerable all over again.

Exactly how Shaun must feel.

She'd let him down. She could admit it now. What next? He'd left work this afternoon, apparently going straight to the airport for his flight to Adelaide. Talking to him, apologising and telling him what he wanted to know, was going to have to wait until he got back. Whenever that was. It was going to seem like forever. Phoning wasn't right. She had to do it face-to-face. Hopefully then he might feel comfortable with talking about his problems. Because they both needed to be honest with each other.

On Saturday, Shaun stood beside Larry, one of his close friends, and watched his sister holding Larry's hands as they exchanged their vows. It brought tears to his eyes to see Joy so happy, something that had been missing in his bright, bubbly little sister for years. After an abusive relationship, she'd sworn she would never again set herself up to be vulnerable to any man, and here she was marrying his friend.

Larry was an emergency doctor at Adelaide Hospital. When Joy moved over here to get away from her ex, Shaun had set them up for a date. Voilà, here they stood, looking beyond happy.

'You could have it too,' Joy had said last night. 'If I can do it, then so can you. You just have to stop hanging on to the past so fiercely.'

'Yeah, right,' he'd retorted. But seeing these two so happy, the thought crossed his mind that maybe his sister had a point. He'd tried but had given in too quickly. Within weeks of returning to Christchurch, his life had started changing. The job was similar to most others, yet he felt he fitted in better at Christchurch General. He didn't spend his time looking for reasons to leave. Until it all went belly up with Nikki. Spending time with the family was awesome. Throw in the house and he'd made progress. All that was left to finish the list was Nikki. Not any woman. Nikki. She'd won him over without trying. His heart was hers to do with as she saw fit. She could break it in one move, or she could love him back and make him the happiest man on the planet.

If he let her. He had to. There was no other way.

'Ladies and gentlemen, girls and boys, I announce Larry and Joy husband and wife. Hip hooray.'

Everyone was on their feet, clapping and calling out congratulations. Kids began running around in circles, laughing loudly.

The waiters were bringing around trays with glasses of champagne.

Shaun waited until no one was talking to Joy and moved in to hug her. 'I am so happy for you, sis. I really am.'

She planted a big kiss on his chin. 'So am I.'

He waited for the dig about sorting his own life out, but it didn't come.

Instead she said, 'I hear you turned down Larry's offer of a job here.'

'I did.' When he'd gone into the ED where his mate worked, he hadn't felt the spark of anticipation at a new job that was normal and knew he was returning home. Home. That was the thing. Christchurch was home. 'I didn't want to be there. I like the position I've got.'

'Sounds positive. Sorry, but I'd better keep moving around.'

'Go for it. This is your and Larry's day.'

'Thanks to you for introducing us.'

They were a perfect match. But what about him and Nikki?

Shaun had spent every free moment since that night they'd argued thinking about Nikki and asking himself if he was wasting an opportunity to tick that final requirement to be at home and completely happy. Opening up and talking about Liam's death would've been hard to do but also would've shown how hurt and vulnerable he was, something he didn't know how to do. It might've lightened his vulnerability. His family understood the pressure he'd put himself under by blaming himself for not being able to save Liam when in reality it had been impossible, but they never actually talked about it with him. If he wanted to become part of Nikki's life, then he had to toughen up, and take it on the chin if she didn't understand why he'd felt he'd let Liam down.

Though he doubted Nikki would think he had done anything wrong that day in the plane. She'd more likely fully understand why he'd been so hurt over losing Liam. She'd been hurt too and knew how hard it was to move on. Couples had to share their feelings, their fears and delights, their pain and joy, not avoid them.

'Looks like you're thinking too much.' Larry was handing him another glass of champagne.

He hadn't realised he'd drunk the first one. 'I'd better go easy.'

Larry smirked. 'It's our wedding. You will enjoy yourself.'

'You've only been married moments, and already you sound like my sister.'

Larry laughed, sounding happier than Shaun could remember him ever being. 'They say love is blind.'

Ping, it was like a bell had gone off in his head. He was blind. He'd fallen for Nikki fast when he knew little about her, and suddenly he made a decision. He didn't want to miss out on trying to make it work between them. Damn it, he'd get down on bended knee if that's what it took to make her give him a chance. 'You know what, you're right.'

'When aren't I?' Larry chuckled. 'Don't tell Joy I said that.'

'You owe me.'

'You won't change your mind about coming over here for that job?'

'Nope.' Not even if he didn't win over Nikki. He was going home to Christchurch. It was the right place for him, and everything had been slotting into place making him more comfortable by the week when he wasn't overthinking it. 'I'm sticking to the plan.' Larry knew what he was trying to do, and Shaun suspected the job offer was his way of toughening him up.

Larry clapped him on the shoulder. 'Good. Now looks like I've got to go get some photos taken. Beats me why we have to do this, but if Joy's happy, then so am I.'

'Yeah, right. I can already see a framed picture of the two of you on the lounge wall in your apartment.'

If he had a photo of Nikki on his phone, he'd be taking it out now and looking at her. He accepted he loved her. He missed her so much it hurt bigtime. Would she give him a second chance when he'd hurt her? Face it, he'd kept her at arm's length too long and now might have lost her for good. They'd been too busy getting to know each other without giving anything away about themselves, which seemed unreal but in their case was true. Forget the list. This was about them and love and making a future together. He didn't care about anything else right now, only Nikki.

Monday night and the sun hadn't quite set, though darkness wasn't far away. Spring was inching closer. Her favourite season when the daffodils flowered in the park and the trees started to bud. Not that the air was much warmer, but it was a start. Nikki walked fast around the perimeter of Hagley Park. It was her second lap, and she felt good.

If she didn't think about Shaun.

Hard to do when he hung out in the back of her mind all the time, popping up to the front whenever she wasn't involved with patients. Annoying at the very least. She wasn't thinking how he affected her so much. It was too raw and too close to her heart. She had to stay in remote mode to get through this, and get through it she would. She'd done it before. She could do it again.

She had to, for her sanity. But this time she wasn't going into a funk and refusing to get out among other people when it came to dating. It was past time to move on and get a real life—the one she'd dreamed of and thought she'd had with Brett. Her strides lengthened. Decision made. She couldn't waste any more time wondering why everything had gone so wrong with Shaun. That was part of life.

When she reached her car, she checked her phone, but no messages from Shaun. As if there would be. She was supposed to be getting over him. Yeah, right. At least she was thinking about doing it.

On the way home, she swung by the Thai take-away shop and picked up an order of green curry, plus a chicken satay to reheat for tomorrow's dinner. Easy as. Cooking for one got to be a chore at times. Most of the time, she admitted with a wry smile. Brett used to say she should get a kitchen maid considering how much effort she put into cooking. Her argument was that being female didn't automatically make her a great cook. He never had an answer for that.

As she turned into her street, the car's headlights lit up a vehicle parked outside her house. A black SUV. Shaun. Wasn't he meant to come home tomorrow? What did he want? Come to tell her he was moving to South Australia? He might as well have waited until tomorrow at work when he could tell everyone. She didn't need a special visit.

Parking in front of her garage, she sucked in a deep breath and reminded herself she was not going to let him into her heart any longer. He was history before he'd been much else. Gathering up the takeaways and her handbag, she got out of the car and locked it, glad for the automatic lighting that came on when she drove in. Then, serious face on, she turned to look at the man walking up her driveway and waited. Her heart rate had lifted, and she had no idea to slow it down other than remain determined to get through whatever this was about without giving in to the love filling her at the sight of Shaun.

'Hello, Nikki.' He stopped and watched her as though waiting for a reaction of any sort.

She only had one. Wrong, she did have reactions that wanted to burst free, only she was keeping those to herself. She couldn't rush up and wrap her arms around him, hold him like she never wanted to let him go, because she wouldn't. 'Hello, Shaun.'

Something was bothering him. He was watching her with an intensity she hadn't seen before. It was hard not to ask what was up, but he didn't like personal questions. This was how she protected herself. She waited.

'Have I come at an inopportune time?' he asked.

'No.'

'I need to talk to you, explain a few things. How we parted last week.' He paused. 'How we stopped getting along so easily—' Another pause. 'It's been hard not seeing you.'

She waited to see where this was going, ignoring the glimmer of hope tapping at her heart.

'I haven't been totally open with you.'

'Nor have I with you.' She shivered. The temperature was dropping now that the sun had disappeared, but her skin was tight. 'Come inside.'

'Thanks.' He followed her in quietly, not saying anything else.

Awkward. Nikki placed the takeaways on the bench and her bag on the table. The silence grew, and in the end she had to say something or lose her cool. 'How was Adelaide?'

He stood at the end of the counter, watching her. 'That's why I'm here.'

So he was leaving Christchurch. Plonking her backside on a stool at the kitchen island, she studied him. He looked tired, and worried, and sad all in one. She let go the hold she had on her emotions. He was too special for her to ignore his pain. 'What's going on, Shaun?'

'First, I'm not here for sympathy. I need to explain what makes me tick so you might understand me a little.'

Was he saying they might have a future together? Or was she getting ahead of herself? That was more likely. But her heart wasn't very good at doing as she told it. 'Go on.'

His wide chest rose as he drew a breath. 'I went

across for my sister's wedding, and seeing her so happy brought me to tears.' He gave her a wobbly smile. 'Yes, I am capable of crying.'

'Who isn't?'

'Joy was in an abusive relationship until a couple of years ago when one day she got up, packed her bags and walked out of the house never to return. It took a lot of guts. She never once considered going back despite the threats the guy made.'

'Now she's moved on and is happy.' *Like I want to be.* With this man if he'd have her.

'Yes, with one of my friends. But that's not what I came to tell you. At least not entirely.' He was struggling, not used to being open about himself.

'Would you like a glass of wine?' It might help him relax a bit and get whatever was bothering him off his chest.

'I'd love one.'

When she placed two glasses on the counter, he sat down opposite her. 'Thanks.'

Taking a sip, she waited. There was nothing she could think of to say to help him overcome whatever was holding him back. If she apologised for her own mistakes now, he might stop what he was trying to say.

His glass was turning back and forwards in his fingers. 'Seeing Joy so happy woke me up to what I could have if I only let go what's been holding me back since Liam died. She made sure

I knew I was wasting time worrying about being vulnerable again. She's right. I have been dodging around what's happened.' He paused and took a mouthful of wine.

'What would that be?' she asked quietly, still not sure where this was going but feeling more and more on edge. She wanted to help him, but she didn't know how and wouldn't until he told her everything.

'You know my friend, Liam, had a cardiac arrest while he was flying us back from Wellington in a small plane. I knew nothing about flying, but I'm a doctor. I know what to do when someone has a heart attack. Except there was no room to lie him out and do CPR, and if there had been, there'd have been no one at the controls to fly the plane.'

'You've blamed yourself ever since.' This was deeper than what she'd read, because it was Shaun telling her what happened.

'It probably sounds OTT, but yes I have. Not all the time, but often. At the time, I had to make a decision and figured getting Liam home to his family in one piece was more important than trying to manage compressions when I knew he was dead. I desperately wanted to do them. Instead I got on the radio and called for help. Liam had shown me how to keep a plane flying straight and level, even how to bring it lower, but in the circumstances, it all felt near impossible. Someone in the control tower who had a private pilot's licence talked me through keeping the plane level until an instructor came across from the nearby aero club and talked me down. It wasn't a great landing, but at least we made it without further problems.'

She couldn't help herself. She reached for his free hand. 'I don't know how you did that.'

'I don't either.' He took another gulp of wine. 'But it only got harder. I was married to Liam's sister, Amy. We were both devastated over what had happened to Liam and struggled to support each other while dealing with our own grief. Then there was her family. They never blamed me for what happened, and I know they were right, but I felt so guilty for not saving him. In the end, it got too much for Amy and me, and we agreed to go our separate ways.'

'So you've been married.' Somehow she wasn't surprised. It added to his reasons for holding back from telling her everything. 'You lost a lot that day.' After squeezing his hand, she let go to give him space.

'I did. Our marriage break-up coming on top of Liam's death made me vulnerable and therefore self-protective. I haven't let anyone in since. Until now. Meeting you has made me open my eyes and really see how I've withdrawn from living life to the full. I'm vulnerable and scared, and because of that, I've hurt you. I'm so sorry.'

Her heart slowed. *Here it comes.* He was going to say he couldn't trust himself with a new relationship.

'The thing is, Nikki—' Again that sexy chest lifted. 'I've fallen in love with you. I really, truly love you, and I want you to know that. I'm sorry I avoided talking about myself earlier, but—'

Nikki was off her stool and stepping between his knees. 'Stop right there, Shaun. We've both held back.' *He loves me.* 'I didn't tell you how I felt about Brett playing around behind my back, how vulnerable that made *me*. I haven't mentioned how hard it was growing up with an egotistical father making us constantly move homes and schools, having to make new friends all the time. I gave you the basics because the rest was too hard to talk about. I laid my heart on the line once, and after how Brett treated me, I've been afraid to repeat that mistake.' *He loves me.* 'Though since meeting you, I've decided being alone is more than lonely. It's ridiculous. I still dream about having a family with the man I give my heart to. You, Shaun. I love you. I think I started falling for you that day in ED when you had my back with the media.'

She couldn't say any more. Not only because of the tears blocking her throat but because Shaun had her head in his hands and was kissing her so gently she wanted to cry—if she wasn't already.

He drew back a fraction. 'Darling Nikki.

You're everything I want. You're one amazing lady, and I love you so much it hurts at times.'

She had to kiss him better.

An hour later, they lay in each other's arms in bed, smiling non-stop. 'Wow,' Nikki whispered.

'Yes, wow. That's the way to start a serious relationship.' Shaun brushed a kiss on her forehead.

Pushing up onto her elbow, Nikki gazed at him. 'Serious relationship? You mean that, don't you?'

He sat up and took her hands in his. 'Yes, sweetheart, I do. To the point that I have to ask— Will you marry me, Nikki Marlow?'

Her heart was beating out of time. 'Y-yes. Absolutely yes, Shaun Elliott.' She'd be Mrs Nikki Elliott. Woo-hoo.

Their kiss was long and deep and filled with all the love they had in them to give.

I'm getting married, Nikki hummed to herself. *To the most amazing man I've ever known.* Life couldn't get better than that.

'I have something else to put to you,' Shaun said.

'What's that?'

'Would you be happy to move into my house with me and make it our home?'

She loved her cottage, but if Shaun was ready to move on from his past and settle down, the least she could do was be there at his side in all ways possible. She'd held back about herself, and this would help make up for that as she moved forward with the love of her life. 'Absolutely.'

'It doesn't mean you get to make all the decisions about the colour scheme and furniture,' he said with a grin.

'We'll see about that.' She laughed. She really couldn't have cared less about any of that right now. All that mattered was she loved Shaun and he loved her back. 'We're getting married. Woo-hoo.'

'That we are.' And he kissed her again. And again.

* * * * *

If you enjoyed this story, check out these other great reads from Sue MacKay

Parisian Surgeon's Secret Child
Wedding Date with the ER Doctor
Brooding Vet for the Wallflower
Healing the Single Dad Surgeon

All available now!

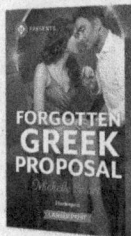

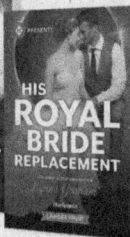

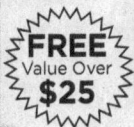

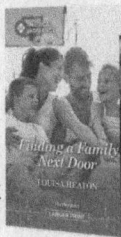

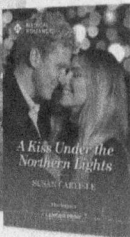